Acclaim for *Rhythms of the Game: The Link Between Musical and Athletic Performance*

"Watching Pedro Martinez mixing pitches and changing speeds, 'composing' a mound masterpiece–most opponents gnashed their teeth and muttered curses. But Bernie Williams saw and appreciated something else–the similarities between a pitcher like Pedro and the inspired riffs of a great jazz musician. This understanding has informed and elevated Williams' performance, both as a player and a musician. Here he takes us inside his two worlds."

–Bob Costas

"A book written with the sound and the silence of people who know by experience the rhythm of the right brain and its role in excellence. This book is not just about the marvels of the relationship between music and baseball; it is about the mysteries of human potential."

–Tim Gallwey, author of *The Inner Game of Tennis*

"Bernie Williams introduced me to his parallel universe in 2009 while I was shooting a feature on him for ESPN. He was out of the majors, but training to play in the World Baseball Classic for his native Puerto Rico while pursuing his music degree at SUNY Purchase. Sitting in on the final edit session for his current album, *Moving Forward*, I watched Bernie agonize over every excruciating detail, ensuring his latest musical work would embody the dedication and work ethic that made him a Yankees fan favorite. *Rhythms of the Game* meshes Bernie's two passions in a way that enables us all to appreciate how baseball and music are so closely intertwined."

–Bonnie Bernstein, ESPN broadcaster

"A deeper thinker, a classical musician, and a Yankee for life."

–John Sterling, play-by-play
radio announcer for the New York Yankees

"You can almost hear the slow jazz tune playing in his head as he's going around the field."

—Sweeny Murti, WFAN Yankee beat reporter

"Was Bernie Williams a musician trapped in a ballplayer's body, or was it the other way around? Dave and Bob tapped into his mind, and the three of them have delivered a gem of a book here."

—Marty Appel, former Yankees public relations director, and author of *Munson, The Life and Death of a Yankee Captain*

*To Marybeth .Thanks for everything !!.*

# Rhythms of the Game

## The Link Between Musical and Athletic Performance

by
Bernie Williams, Dave Gluck, and Bob Thompson

With a Foreword by Paul Simon

Hal Leonard Books
An Imprint of Hal Leonard Corporation

Published in 2011 by Hal Leonard Books
An Imprint of Hal Leonard Corporation
7777 West Bluemound Road
Milwaukee, WI 53213

Trade Book Division Editorial Offices
33 Plymouth St., Montclair, NJ 07042

Permissions can be be found on page 205, which constitutes an extension of this copyright page.
Printed in the United States of America

Book design by Damien Castaneda

Library of Congress Cataloging-in-Publication Data

Williams, Bernie, 1968-
  Rhythms of the game : the link between musical and athletic performance / by Bernie
    Williams, Dave Gluck, and Bob Thompson.
      p. cm.
  Includes bibliographical references.
  ISBN 978-1-4234-9947-3 (hardcover)
  1. Music and sports. 2. Music--Performance. 3. Baseball--Songs and music--History and
    criticism. 4. Sports--Physiological aspects. I. Gluck, Dave. II. Thompson, Bob (Robert
    F.), 1960- III. Title.
  ML3916.W55 2011
  780'.0796--dc22

                    2011013718


www.halleonardbooks.com

*To our parents*

# Contents

# Foreword

I was standing in centerfield at the old Yankee Stadium talking with Bernie Williams. It was the 23rd of April 1999, the day the Yankees were to celebrate the legendary Joe DiMaggio with the unveiling of a monument in his honor. My purpose, standing there in center, was to do a sound check for a performance of "Mrs. Robinson" at the pregame ceremony. Bernie was strolling toward the clubhouse to begin his warm-ups, and we stood together gazing at the stadium's three-tiered grandeur from the perspective of Mantle, DiMaggio, and . . . Williams.

"How do you control your nerves in a situation like today's?" Williams asked me.

"How do you come to bat in a World Series game and block out everything but the spin of a baseball traveling at ninety-five miles per hour?"" was my counter-question to him.

The answer to both queries is the same: you're outside looking in, inside your own world of calm but heightened awareness. The world of "the zone."

Williams recalled his eleventh-inning at bat in the '96 ALCS as a zone-like experience. Playing the field in the top of the inning, he remembered thinking that he would either walk or hit a home run in his next plate appearance. In the on-deck circle in the bottom of the eleventh, his concentration on the pitcher, Randy Myers, was so intense that he felt he could intuit the pitch before it was thrown. When he came to bat, the baseball looked as big as a beach ball. He hit a home run.

Elite athletes and gifted musicians have a lot in common—years of training and thousands of hours of practice, an innate inclination toward excellence, musicians are often cited as having "great ears" and athletes are blessed with unusually strong and flexible bodies, and both professions share a sense of rhythm and flow. But within the constellation of similarities, none is more mysterious than those rare but memorable periods of time, or timelessness, called "the zone," a place of focused attention, improved muscle control, and a reduction of anxiety.

Williams remembered the '98 Yankees, a team that won 125 games on their way to a World Championship, as a group of players that spent the entire season in "the zone," as though the energy of individual players could suffuse an entire clubhouse. When I recount the amount of remarkable and enduring music that was produced between the years 1966 and 1970, I'm inclined to see it as a similar phenomenon. Consider that the Beach Boys' *Pet Sounds*, the Beatles' *Sgt. Pepper*, Dylan's *Blonde on Blonde*, Hendrix's *Are You Experienced*, Simon and Garfunkel's *Bridge Over Troubled Water*, Aretha Franklin's *Respect*, and Carole King's *Tapestry* were all produced in this four-year span and one suspects that the atmosphere was charged with a "zone-like" energy.

Standing in centerfield that spring afternoon, I was aware that the stadium was packed. I could see the Yankee players on the top step of the dugout and I heard the public-address announcer speak my name. Everything seemed to slow down. I was completely focused on the sound in my earpiece, the slap of the strings against the neck of the guitar, the sound of my voice singing a slower, more mournful "Where have you gone Joe DiMaggio?"

In the magic of "the zone," the world changes shape to suit the will of its inhabitants.

– Paul Simon

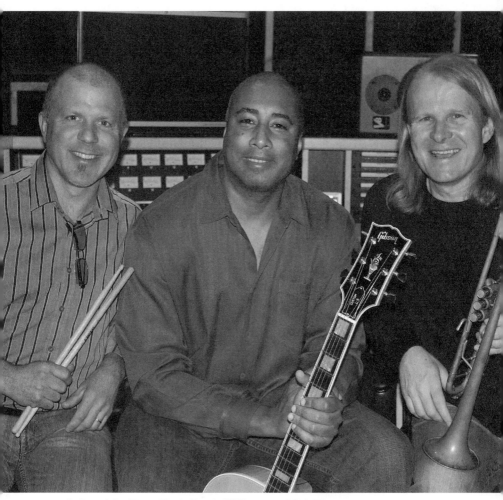
Left to right: Dave Gluck, Bernie Williams, and Bob Thompson.

# Preface: Tinkers to Evers to Chance

The first question people ask us is, "How did the three of you end up writing a book together?" We're not exactly "Tinkers to Evers to Chance"–that amazing Chicago Cubs trio from the early 1900s that perfected the modern double play. Sadly, only one of us has ever hit a baseball farther than 250 feet (but did so quite frequently over the course of sixteen years). Even more sadly, only one of us has a perfect hitting record, striking out continuously in two years of little league (that would be Bob, a left-handed catcher who batted .000 but managed a few walks, so he knows what first base feels like). Our commonality, however, is that baseball and music were the "star dirt" of our childhoods, and has carried us through adulthood, in one way or another.

But before we tell you the story of how *Rhythms of the Game* came to be written and co-authored by the three of us, we need to run around the bases with you first, and explain a few phrases never before uttered by any musician or ballplayer we know–phrases like "narrative mode" and "grammatical person" (not to be confused with grammatical persona–which is embodied in Yogi Berra, a master at writing grammatically correct sentences that leave you scratching your head–sentences like, "I didn't really say everything I said"). In this book, we say a lot, but not everything we say is said by all of us, and some of what's said in this book is said by none of us. Yogi's rubbed off on us a bit. Let us explain.

There are a number of books with three co-authors, but we've yet to find a book with three co-authors writing both separately in their own narrative voice as well as collectively as co-authors. Bob Woodward and Carl Bernstein did so rather successfully in their book, *All the President's Men*, about the Watergate scandal. It was a perfect narrative double play. With *Rhythms of the Game*, however, we're attempting a never-before-seen narrative triple play. Three authors, three voices, one book. By necessity, that means we're occasionally running from first to second to third (person, that is–not base).

The majority of the book is written in first person plural ("we"–as in the three of us), alternating with the first person singular ("I"). In the case of the latter ("I"), we've taken great pains to be sure you know which of us is talking (and kindly note that, regrettably, only one of us has played major league baseball, much less win four World Series. You should have no problem figuring out when that co-author is at bat).

Sometimes we'll relate a concept in the second person ("you" or "they") to help you, the aspiring musician or athlete, better grasp that concept. There are also a number of sidebars in the book contributed by experts in the field (or on the stage) and the authorship of those is clearly noted.

Finally, on a few occasions, we'll talk about ourselves in the third person (substituting "Dave, Bob, and Bernie" in place of "we"). Talking in the third person when referring to oneself is usually reserved for either European royalty or the exhausted parents of toddlers (as in, "Daddy's trying to write this book now, so could you kids stop throwing baseballs at him?"). Now that we've covered all the grammatical bases, here's the backstory. Follow the ball closely.

Bob and Dave have worked together for many years. Both were touring musicians–and in 1993, were co-founders of a six-piece eclectic jazz/classical group called Rhythm and Brass, which toured the planet (and continues to do so). Bob left that group in 1995 to move to Europe and run a music company–but the last project the two worked on together with Rhythm and Brass was a collaboration with the Rochester Philharmonic. Members of the group were to appear as soloists with the orchestra, and as a bonus, the orchestra commissioned composer Fred Sturm to write a piece for the group and the Philharmonic to premiere in May of that year. Fred, an avid baseball fan, composed a nine-movement work called "A Place Where It Would Always Be Spring," which utilized some of the great poems and writings about baseball as spoken text. Former New York Yankee Tony Kubek was the narrator at the premiere, and Hall of Famer Dave Winfield picked up where Tony left off and has been narrating the work ever since.

Dave continued touring with Rhythm and Brass while Bernie was belting out hit after hit, acquiring four new rings. Bob spent years in Europe without his beloved Yankees–his only connection to the game was via sporadic Armed Forces Radio broadcasts. Feeling homesick, he returned to the USA as a free agent, started The Baseball Music Project in 2006 with Dave Winfield, and signed on for a two-year stint as dean of music at the State University of New York at Purchase College, where coincidentally Dave had become a professor of studio composition (a program that's produced singer-songwriters the likes of Moby and Regina Spektor). That same year, Bernie ended his amazing sixteen-year career with the Yankees. Bernie stopped by Bob's office on a cold, snow-covered day in December 2007, seeking to hone his guitar and composition skills so that he could focus full-time on his music career. Bob introduced Bernie to Dave, and by the end of the meeting, Bernie enrolled in a myriad of courses that would help him prepare for his next album.

Dave became Bernie's composition teacher and Bob became Bernie's dean. Dave worked with Bernie on some of the songs for the new album–and the title cut, "Moving Forward," came out of those composition lessons. Bernie reciprocated and gave Dave's son Julian a coaching session on hitting in Dave's office–and the next day, Dave yelled to Julian before his Little League at bat, "Don't forget what Bernie told ya!" The next pitch resulted in a double.

Bob gave Bernie a copy of a new book he had co-authored, *Baseball's Greatest Hit: The Story of "Take Me Out to the Ball Game,"* and Bernie came back a week later and said, "Hey, Dean Bob! I've got something I want you to hear!" It was Bernie's slow and melancholic version of "Take Me Out to the Ball Game"–his swan song to the game–and it became the final cut on the album *Moving Forward*, which garnered a Latin Grammy nomination. The album was a critical success (and as Bob and Dave will tell you–Bernie is an exceptional musical talent).

The idea for *Rhythms of the Game*, however, grew out of an alumni weekend event, where Bob moderated as Dave and Bernie discussed the parallel mindsets of ballplayers and musicians. We think there's another reason why ballplayers and musicians feel so at home with one another: they speak the same language. Only a batter and a bassoonist can ask interchangeable questions like "Was that pitch low?" or "Is my tempo off?" As we spent more time in both the worlds of baseball and music, it became evident that we had stumbled onto something: baseball and music are indelibly intertwined.

The three of us have spent a lifetime in both worlds–one of us got sidetracked by taking a musically harmonious route playing for the Yankees (but kept his guitar with him while on the road) and two of us spent years as touring musicians (and our baseball gloves were always with us–except possibly in winter). The choice to pursue one career over the other came down to timing, talent, circumstances, and personal choice (in the talent area, clearly, one of us excelled early on, on the field, while the other two excelled early on up on the stage).

The three of us share uncanny and parallel creative mindsets, and regardless of whether that creativity plays out on the field or on the stage, the mindset is the same, the approach is the same, the fundamentals are the same, and there is, at least in our minds, no separating the two. Baseball has informed how we play music, and for one of us, music informed how the game was played.

We kept up the conversations–hung out, watched reruns of old Yankees games–and even went to one together. The more we talked to musicians and ballplayers, the more the parallels became evident. *Rhythms of the Game* is a natural outpouring of our conversations the past three years.

We're all now full-time professional musicians–performing, composing, touring, producing, recording, and–writing. But baseball is always there. Bernie is now enjoying a post-baseball second-career renaissance as a musician, and his artistry continues to grow by leaps and bounds. Bob and Dave joke that if Bernie's career continues at this pace, his Wikipedia entry might just end with the footnote, "Some fans may remember he also played major league baseball."

# Introduction

∾ ∾ ∾

*Baseball's time is seamless and invisible, a bubble within which players move at exactly the same pace and rhythms as all their predecessors.*
— ROGER ANGELL, *THE SUMMER GAME*

The interrelationship between music and sport is storied and ancient. In fact, the idea was a pillar of society and philosophy long before baseball was invented. Very long before.

Around 380 BC, the Greek philosopher Plato wrote in *The Republic* about the idealized society as having a "united influence of music and sport" where its people "mingle music with sport in the fairest of proportions." In Greek civilization, music and sport were viewed as synonymous, complimentary, and, above all, both necessary for a person's full development and education. The Greek view was that sport and music went together–their sum greater than their parts. If Plato showed up today at a contentious school budget meeting, with parents jockeying over whether sports or the arts should be cut, he'd argue that both the marching band and the baseball team should be saved (but might suggest they both put off getting new uniforms). In Plato's world, it made no sense to have one without the other. We like Plato.

In modern times, music and sport have shared an entertaining and strategic bond. Professional team sports usually involve music on some basic level–whether it's entertainment (singing "Take Me Out to the Ball Game" during a seventh-inning stretch) or strategic (blasting Metallica's "Enter Sandman" to psychologically intimidate the visiting team at Yankee Stadium when Mariano Rivera enters from the center-field bullpen–not that Mo needs any musical assistance, thank you). And let's not forget the Super Bowl halftime show (pure entertainment) or the ear-numbing roar of 10,000 "vuvuzelas" at a FIFA World Cup (pure intimidation).

Beyond music's entertainment and "strategic" value, the fields of music and sports psychology have proliferated in the last half-century, leading to a number of studies and books, most notably Tim Gallwey's *The Inner Game of Tennis* (followed by Barry Green's *The Inner Game of Music*) and the writings and teachings of sports and music psychologist Dr. Don Greene (who has contributed to this book). The study of music's effect on peak-level sports performance has proliferated as well–from examining how music increases endurance in marathon runners to improving a rowing team's sprint performance level, as well as decreasing reaction times among tennis players.

Beyond this scientific research, there has been scant exploration linking the creative processes of music (such as intuition, nuance, rhythm, composition, improvisation, and artistry) to sports, which has left us with several unanswered questions: Do musical rhythms play a roll in a sport like baseball? Is there a link between the creative process of a musician and the creative process of a pitcher? Is there a point where extreme athleticism ceases to be sport–and evolves into art? Can a deeper understanding of music and its amalgam of sounds, timbres, rhythms, and structures assist the athlete attempting to improve his or her game? What, if any, are the parallel creative mindsets of elite athletes and musicians?

More broadly, how can musicians and athletes develop better practice and performance skills, and are there lessons to be learned from one discipline that are applicable to the other? Finally, does a sport such as baseball have anything to teach the aspiring musician? We examine these questions and explore the nexus of athleticism and music, specifically through the sport that has the closest kinship to music–baseball.

The structure of *Rhythms of the Game*, as we mentioned in the preface, is a combination of collective narratives (the three of us writing as one voice) and single narratives (where one of us takes the microphone and relates a key concept). Interspersed between these narratives are a series of sidebars from experts in the field. The chapters in this book are divided into three parts.

Chapters 1–3 lay the groundwork–the shared history of music and baseball, and the similarities between a performer onstage and a ballplayer on the field. A universal commonality between professional musicians and pro athletes is that they must "perform" in public. We believe peak performance is a rarified space, independent of the medium (music or sport), where a bat and a baton are simply props–canvasses upon which artists create, intuit, and conjure those magical moments of greatness.

A crucial component in this book is that one of us was able to achieve a level of elite performance in *both* sports and music. It is not often that musicians and athletes have an artistic interpreter–one who can translate the experience of hitting a major league postseason home run in extra innings into performing at an exceptionally high level on the concert stage in front of a packed house. In addition, we have our own performance-enhancement specialist, Dr. Don Greene, waiting in the on-deck circle. Don's worked with the U.S. Olympic team, the Texas Rangers, the Cal Berkeley baseball team, and taught at the Juilliard School, in addition to working with innumerable professional musicians around the world. His sidebars throughout the book illuminate the science and psychology behind the artistic and performance concepts we discuss.

Chapters 4–13 deal specifically with the parallel mindsets of ballplayers and musicians, exploring the psychology, strategy, and ingredients needed to perform at an elite level. We begin with "The Matrix Moment" (a hyper-focused state under enormous pressure where an athlete or musician is able to create that "genius" moment) and work backward, dissecting that moment through concepts related to intuition, anticipation, artistry, composition, mental and rhythmic acuity, along with developing focus and mental endurance.

We explore in these chapters the mind of "the zone"–and the similarities between a Paul Simon performing at a high level in front of 500,000 supportive fans or a Derek Jeter performing at the same level at Fenway in front of 37,000 jeering ones. We explore the notion of strategy, as in composing a game (through the mind of the great Pedro Martinez) or improvising a solo (through the mind of the legendary John Coltrane). We also explore a seldom discussed concept related to achieving peak performance in music and sport: reducing variables, along with concepts for increasing one's mental focus and toughness. These chapters collectively lead to the chapter "The Art of Performing," where we explore how to "practice performing."

Chapters 14–22 deal primarily with philosophy (the philosophy of competition, failure, teamwork, leadership–and even parenting the young musician or athlete) along with practical matters (fundamentals, mechanics, and slumps). These chapters take a step back from the field or the stage, providing context for the first two sections of the book.

The Postscript, titled "The Sound Track of Summer," includes a few fun sidebars on everything from our favorite concerts to the "musical" psychology behind jeering at ball games to a contribution from Tim Wiles at the Baseball Hall of Fame, titled "The Soundtrack of Summer." At the back of the book, you'll find an extensive bibliography that can serve as the leadoff hit to further exploring the topics we discuss.

It's our hope that you, the reader–whether you're an aspiring athlete, musician, or simply a devoted fan–will come away with a deeper understanding and appreciation of the parallel mindsets of athletes and musicians. For the fan of music and/or sports, we believe this book will enhance the experience of watching elite musicians and athletes perform. For those readers aspiring to a career on the field or onstage, we believe this book will help you in developing your craft.

The baseball-writing luminary Roger Angell once wrote, "Baseball's time is seamless and invisible, a bubble within which players move at exactly the same pace and rhythms as all their predecessors." The themes outlined in this book are universal and timeless too–while players change and musical styles evolve, the rhythms of the game have remained constant.

# AFFECTIVE ARTISTRY

........................................................................................................

by Bob Thompson

........................................................................................................

The lack of exploration into the parallel creative and artistic realms of sports and music stems from the fact that—as much as one might research the psychology of music or sports—the artistic "affect" of sports and music (that which makes it creative, singular, and personal) lives primarily in a nonverbal world. There exists a plethora of articles and discussions on the genius of Beethoven's *Eroica* symphony, as well as Don Larsen's perfect game in the 1956 World Series. However, explaining genius is not the same thing as experiencing it. True artistry is part mystery—you can't quite put your finger on what it is that makes it so. It can't be fully explained or completely understood—and perhaps it never was intended to be. However, it can be experienced.

Take, for instance, the Beatles. The three of us believe that the Beatles were pure genius. Two of us have even taught courses on the Beatles—analyzing, dissecting, and discerning what went into their genius—but our feeble attempts ultimately fail. The only way to truly experience the genius of the Fab Four is simply to listen to it.

Similarly, sports analysts have attempted to dissect the combinative artistry of Omar Vizquel and Roberto Alomar and their ability to make mind-boggling double plays. But again, the attempts ultimately fail—Vizquel and Alomar were pure genius, and the only way to truly experience that genius is simply to observe it.

Part of the learning process for both creative athletes and musicians is acquiring the ability to deepen the experiential encounters with those rare artistic "genius moments"—the Yo-Yo Ma moment, the Gretzky moment, the Miles Davis moment, or the Michael Jordan moment—and learn from them.

# 1
# Time Is of the Essence

*The rhythms break,*
*More varied and subtle*
*Than any kind of dance;*
*Movement speeds up*
*Or lags.*

*The ball goes out*
*In sharp and angular drives,*
*Or long, slow ones,*
*Comes in again*
*Controlled*
*And under aim;*

*The players wheel or sprint,*
*Race,*
*Stoop,*
*Slide,*
*Halt,*

*Shift imperceptibly to new positions,*
*Watching the signs,*
*According to the batter,*
*The score,*
*The inning.*
*Time is of the essence . . .*

–Rolfe Humphries, "Polo Grounds"

Imagine a perfect September evening in New York City, game-time temperature is sixty-eight degrees, skies are clear, humidity is low. It's a calm night–but there's fever in the air. The hottest tickets in town on this evening are at two of the cities' greatest arenas.

At 32nd Street and 7th Avenue in Manhattan, the stage crew is going through the final preparations for the first of three shows that will rock New York to its core. This is no ordinary city (as any New Yorker will tell you) and tonight will be no ordinary show.

Outside, traffic snarls and slows to a crawl while the sidewalks around the arena fill with eager fans waiting for the doors to open. New York is always loud and noisy, but even the most cynical and jaded New Yorker passing by would admit this is not a typical night in Manhattan.

The mood inside the empty arena couldn't be more extreme. On a dark stage with only house lights on, the lighting director is conferring with the stage manager, pointing up at the banks of lights secured to towers of rigging, all deliberately pitched and set in place to illuminate the elaborate stage. It took the crew (which numbered close to 150), twenty-four nonstop hours to unload the twenty-eight semi-tractor trailers, hang 200 motor points, set up 2,000 feet of lighting and scenic trussing, lay two miles of power and control cables, hang a hundred state-of-the-art audio speakers suspended in massive arrays around the elaborate, multi-tiered 4,000-square-foot stage, along with another hundred speaker stacks, subwoofers, and monitors at floor level that will turn the audience on its head.

While the lighting director finishes up with the stage manager, the sound engineer is somewhere out in the darkness of the arena among the rows and rows of seats, surrounded by racks of audio gear, hunched over a mixing board, reviewing changes made during the sound check that took place but an hour ago. As the lighting director and stage manager leave the stage, the sound engineer is alone and takes note of the moment: the arena is empty but the air has become electric. Something special is going to happen tonight.

Nine miles to the north, at the corner of 161st and River Avenue, the grounds crew is going through similar motions, making final preparations for a three-day showdown at the greatest stage in the Bronx. The gates open earlier here, and fans are already filling the seats as the managers confer with their trainers and coaches, review their lineups, and make those last-minute game-time decisions. It's a routine that's played out exactly eighty-one times a year in the Bronx—no more, no less.

But tonight is different. The next three days will be different—the Red Sox are in town. And if the Red Sox are in town (as any New York fan will tell you), it's no ordinary night.

Backstage in a dressing room on 32nd Street, the four musicians that form one of the greatest rock 'n' roll bands in history are going over their lineup as well, as the doors to the arena open and crowds pour in. The band backstage can hear the cheers. Just like their counterparts in the Bronx, they too had their own batting practice earlier, which took place in the form of a sound check. They've decided to start the show big. No build up—just hard rock—and the leadoff tune is guaranteed to shake the house.

The leadoff hitter for the home team back in the Bronx comes as no surprise to the opposing manager. Since his rise to the majors, the legendary stadium announcer Bob Sheppard has intoned this shortstop's name and number prior to every home at bat—and Sheppard will continue to do so for as long as this player wears the uniform with the number 2 on his back.

The lead singer back on 32nd and 7th won't get an introduction, however. He doesn't need it. Every soul in the arena knows who he is—they grew up with him. He's rock 'n' roll's first bad boy. Not that Number 2 back in the Bronx needs an introduction either. Every soul in the stadium knows him too—he grew up with them.

Back on 32nd Street, the event is slated to start at 8:00 p.m., and although rock bands are notoriously late in their start times, tonight will be different. Back in the Bronx, a broadcast on network television pushes the usual start time of 7:05 p.m. back an hour. Unbeknownst to the crowd at either stage, the stars have aligned tonight and both events will begin at precisely the same time.

To get the full effect of this particular night in New York, imagine these two events as a split screen on your television—the Bronx on your left, Manhattan on your right.

At precisely the same time, the four musicians that put the *rock* in rock 'n' roll—the Rolling Stones—take the stage amid a frenzied crowd, launching into one of the most recognized guitar vamps on the planet—"Jumpin' Jack Flash"—while nine miles to the north, the most storied major league franchise in history—the New York Yankees—jump from the dugout and take the field. The crowds are in sync, in unison, interchangeable. And they are all screaming. Mick Jagger struts over to the mike as Derek Jeter takes his position at shortstop.

Now turn up the soundtrack from the Garden, mute the volume from the Bronx, and watch and listen. The game is about to begin, Mick Jagger takes the mike, the Yankees are volleying balls across the field, and Keith Richards, Charlie Watts, and Ronnie Wood are locked into an extended vamp. But stay tuned—if you're lucky, an illusion will emerge—and those random volleys across the field won't seem so random after all—in fact, it appears they're choreographed with the precision timing of Cirque du Soleil to Charlie, Ronnie, and Keith jamming. Every rhythm on the field appears to be in sync to the music—even the motion of the players themselves—the windup, the delivery, the throw, the catch—are in sync.

When it happens, it's magical. The music becomes inseparable from the game and the game becomes inseparable from the music—the two are one. You'll be tempted to think your mind is playing tricks on your eyes and ears—but let your mind play on. There's a rhythm to this game. And it was discovered over a century ago.

# 2
# Music of the Sphere

A brief history of music and baseball

*I think there are only three things America will be known for 2,000 years from now when they study this civilization: the Constitution, jazz music, and baseball.*
—GERALD EARLY

*As a kid, before I could play music, I remember baseball being the one thing that could always make me happy.*
—GARTH BROOKS

*I found last winter I played with more emotion. I used to be shy and backward, but those Brooklyn fans cured me of that.*
—EDDIE BASINSKI,
VIOLINIST AND BROOKLYN DODGERS SHORTSTOP, COMMENTING ON HOW
BASEBALL AFFECTED HIS VIOLIN PLAYING WHEN HE RETURNED FROM
PLAYING WITH THE BUFFALO PHILHARMONIC DURING THE OFF-SEASON

Beginning in the late 1800s, a composer and insurance executive from Connecticut by the name of Charles Ives studied the rhythms of baseball. A pitcher and captain of his baseball team in high school, Ives went on to study music at Yale, emerging to become perhaps the most important composer in early twentieth-century America. Ives was baseball's first resident music theorist—studying the inner workings of baseball, the motions, the timings, and the plays. He observed countless games, and given his prowess on the field, began to notice the interplay of music and baseball, and the parallel minds of players and musicians. All these elements of the game—the rhythms and timing—found their way into his music. He even composed a work, "All the Way Around and Back"–that was a musical palindrome depicting the journey of a base runner from first to third base and back again during a foul ball.

One area that particularly peaked Ives's interest (perhaps due to his day job selling insurance) was the notion of risk. Ballplayers take calculated risks–stealing, diving for a ball hit to center to get the final out, throwing a changeup on a 3–2 count. Musicians do too. The Beatles, for example, took a series of risks in their musical development that brought them from the early days of "I Wanna Hold Your Hand" to "A Day in the Life" and the album we know as *Sgt. Pepper.*

Ives saw that ballplayers and musicians were both creative risk takers, but in Ives's mind, ballplayers were truly the risk takers–taking chances every inning, with the risk of failure ever-present, in order to reach a higher plateau. Ives went on to become the most radical American composer of his era–Europeans revered his music, but Americans were slow to appreciate it–and yet it was America's national pastime that instilled in him the need to take musical risks. At the age of seventy-three, he won the Pulitzer Prize in music.

While baseball and music share this level of risk taking, baseball shares something else with music: rhythm. Baseball is indisputably the most musically rhythmic and complex sport invented. It has its ballads, its swing, its salsa–and even its disco. It has its anthems, its medieval chant, and even its own tango between batter and pitcher. There are rhythms to infield pop outs, double plays, line drives, and triples. If you look down on the field from the upper deck during a bases-loaded double to left center, the movements of players on the field appear strangely choreographed–and what can be choreographed can be set to music.

The game's highest level of musical nuance, however, can be found on the mound–a rhythmic tango between batter and pitcher. The rhythm of a pitcher's fastball, slider, curve, changeup, sinker, and cutter all have a distinct tempo and structure that can be musically understood and notated. If you know the tempo of a pitcher's slider and understand it musically, the probability of being in sync with that pitch as you start your swing will be all that much higher.

The languages of baseball and music are interchangeable—musicians on the stage and teams on the field are called by the same name—players. The most common terms in both fields are identical. Think *rhythm, pitch, tempo, time.* If you know and understand this language, you know the game. The jazz musician Wynton Marsalis once said that the highest level of artistry is nuance. Baseball is artistry too—and its nuances, as the poet Rolfe Humphries rightly observed, are "more varied and subtle than any kind of dance."

Apart from the rhythms and nuances of the game, music shares a unique, unparalleled relationship to the sport. More than 2,500 songs have been written about baseball—more than any other sport (and next to love, perhaps more than any other subject). In one rare musical moment, over 1,000 songs were written in just ninety days about just one team (the Hollywood Stars—a Pacific Coast League team—sponsored a three-month songwriting contest in 1954, during which they received over 1,000 entries submitted from thirteen states). The Library of Congress even has a section devoted solely to music about baseball.

When Walter O'Malley told Brooklyn he was taking the Dodgers to Los Angeles, Brooklyn hit back hard with baseball's one and only protest song, "Let's Keep the Dodgers in Brooklyn." When Joe DiMaggio went on a fifty-six-game hitting streak, Les Brown and his Band of Renown cheered with "Joltin' Joe DiMaggio." When Jackie Robinson broke major league's color barrier in 1947, the legendary Count Basie and his band paid tribute with "Did You See Jackie Robinson Hit That Ball?" The "Say Hey Kid," Willie Mays, was celebrated in the song "Say Hey" by The Treniers, and Larry Doby was honored along with Robinson in Brownie McGhee's "Robbie-Doby Boogie."

No other sport has seen such a cross-pollination of musician-ballplayers—Babe Ruth (pianist) to Eddie Basinski (violinist) to Denny McClain (jazz organist) to Bronson Arroyo and Jake Peavy (guitarists), along with ballplayer-musicians from John Philip Sousa to Garth Brooks, to name a few (you can read about more in chapter 23, "The Sound Track of Summer"). Sousa even fielded his own amateur baseball team—and Basinski holds the distinction of being the only major league ballplayer to play in a major orchestra in the same season (the Brooklyn Dodgers and the Buffalo Philharmonic, in 1945).

Music at a ball game is much more than folly: the music played before every at bat aligns with the personality of the player ("Welcome to the Jungle" for Randy Johnson) or the magic of the moment (Mariano Rivera emerging from center field in the ninth inning to Metallica's "Enter Sandman"). The chants and charges are designed to create musical peaks from dull valleys, inspiring the crowd and, hopefully, the home team. In many a ball park, the sounds of a home run—the crack of the bat, the roar of the crowd—are followed by Randy Newman's final theme to that perennial baseball film, *The Natural.*

And in one of the sport's most endearing moments, it's the only game on the planet where—2,430 times each season—the action stops two-thirds through so that ballplayers, fans, and umpires can partake in singing a waltz.

America's first number-one pop hit was a song about a ballplayer—"Slide Kelly Slide!"—written in 1889 in tribute to the dashing Mike King Kelly. There's John Fogerty's "Centerfield" and Terry Cashman's "Talkin' Baseball," Bruce Springsteen's "Glory Days" and Eddie Vedder's "All the Way," "Tessie" by the Dropkick Murphys and "Catfish" by Bob Dylan. No Yankee fan leaves the Bronx without hearing Sinatra's "New York, New York" and no Red Sox fan is truly a member of Red Sox Nation without singing the refrain to Neil Diamond's "Sweet Caroline" at Fenway.

The names of players are not exempt from musical interpretation either—the lyrics to the song "Van Lingle Mungo," by jazz pianist and composer Dave Frishberg, consist of nothing but names of ballplayers past. The American Society of Composers, Authors and Publishers (ASCAP) happily reports that baseball's anthem—"Take Me Out to the Ball

Game"– is played continuously on radio or television some-where in the world 365 days a year, including Christmas and New Year's–but every Chicago Cubs fan will tell you that there is only one true version and Harry Caray is singing it in heaven this very moment.

Abner Doubleday, who was for years widely credited with creating baseball, was in fact a musician, and Henry Chadwick, the "Father of Baseball" and the creator of the box score, was a music teacher and published composer of some fifty songs. Music and baseball share an undercurrent, a language, a connection unlike any between the sports and the arts. The creation of baseball, in its symmetry and de-sign, is inherently rhythmic and musical.

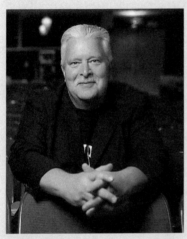

## BEETHOVEN'S NINTH

by Fred Sturm, ASCAP award-winning composer, director of jazz studies at Law-rence University, and artistic director for The Baseball Music Project

Like music, baseball has melody, har-mony, and rhythm. There's melody in the crack of the bat, the slap of the mitt, the ump shouting, "Play ball!" There's harmony in the chatter of infielders and the cheering of the crowd. There's rhythm to one up, one down, two on, two out, and three strikes, three outs.

The Splendid Splinter (Ted Williams) is Horowitz performing Rachmaninoff. Sandy Koufax pitching is Nat King Cole singing "Nature Boy." Willie Mays on base is John Coltrane improvising over "Giant Steps."

Imagine Tchaikovsky's *1812 Overture* accompanying Hank Aaron's 715th home run, Barber's *Adagio for Strings* behind Gehrig's farewell, Beethoven's Ninth in the bottom of the ninth–an *Ode to Joy*–as Bobby Thomson's shot wins the pennant for the Giants, and finally, Handel's *Hallelujah* chorus soar-ing from the rafters of Wrigley Field when my Cubs win another pennant.

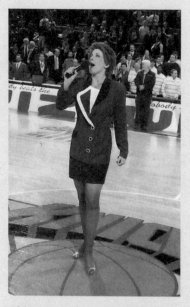

# PASODOBLE

by Suzyn Waldman, radio broadcaster–
New York Yankees, and former Broadway
musical actress

The special ones have that "jazz musician" in them . . . the ability to create what is infinitely special within the finite boundaries of the rules of the game of baseball. That was Bernie Williams—ballplayer, artist, and performer.

Being there from the beginning, it didn't take me long to see the musician in the way Bernie played the game: perhaps a bit unorthodox, listening to his own lyrics and music as he played, but developing into one of the rare few who creates his own moments of greatness. On a baseball field, or on a stage, it's all the same . . . Bernie is a special performer.

Since I was a child, I always thought that baseball at its best had a lyricism and musicality to it. The structure of a symphony or any great piece of music is always the same . . . it's what happens between the staffs of the composition that makes the music special. They all have a beginning, middle, and end . . . they are not all "special." Bernie knew how to brilliantly compose between those lines, and improvise within the structure, with remarkable results. That's what made him special. The brilliant jazz musician performing on the stage of baseball.

One of my favorite memories was Bernie coming into contact with another great jazz musician on the field . . . the pitcher Pedro Martinez. Watching Bernie battle Pedro was like watching two great jazz guitarists go at each other . . . Wes Montgomery and Joe Pass jamming at the Blue Note. The Pedro–Bernie battles were like watching a great *pasodoble* . . . the Spanish musical style played as the matador and his bull meet in the ring, each one trying to best the other. You could feel Bernie's mind going as he stepped out of the box, trying to figure out what Pedro would do next. You could see the little smile on Pedro's face and see his eyes watching Bernie, each one trying to stay one step ahead of the other. At that point, the duels weren't just baseball . . . they were *art*. They were music.

# 3
# Rhythms of the Game

How music influenced my career in major
league baseball

Throughout my musical life in baseball, my guitar has always been with me. I grew up in Puerto Rico, and one of my earliest musical memories was listening to my father play the guitar. He dabbled in it, but I especially remember him playing the traditional *Aguinaldos*–songs often played as part of *Parranda*, a Christmas serenading tradition of Puerto Rico where *Parranda* musicians would stroll from house to house. The music of my childhood began with this wonderful music, played on original instruments such as the *cuatro* (a smaller four-string version of the guitar) and *bordonúa* (bass guitar), along with percussion instruments such the *güiro, maracas*, and *plenaras*.

My family loved listening to music, and I remember my parents playing albums by Trío Los Panchos, a bolero trio. On Saturdays and Sundays, our house was filled with their music. It is impossible to grow up in Puerto Rico and not be influenced by the country's musical heritage–the rich rhythmic styles of *salsa, bomba, plena, seis*, and *danza*. All these musical forms have one thing in common: rhythm. Rhythm was a part of my childhood–and whether I was playing music or baseball–it all flowed from the same deep well called rhythm. It didn't seem very different to me whether I had a guitar in my hand or a bat: the rhythms were the same. Whenever I'd step up to the plate, I could have as well been playing a *pasadoble* (a Spanish dance that depicts the duel between matador and bull, or in my case, between pitcher and batter) with my guitar. It was all about the rhythm.

I started playing guitar when I was seven–and the first

tune I learned was–believe it or not–a TV theme from a scotch whiskey commercial, with Jose Feliciano playing and singing. I never put my guitar down after that. Music was in my life.

In 1977, Billy Martin led the Yankees to their first World Series in sixteen years, in part due to the pitching of Ron Guidry. The fact that Yankees fans now stand and clap when there are two strikes on the opposing batter began with Guidry in 1978, the year in which he recorded a record-breaking eighteen strikeouts in one game. A lesser known fact about Guidry is that he played drums–in the Yankees clubhouse. Guidry had a drum set stored in a storage room off of the clubhouse and only the clubhouse manager and Guidry had the key. During rain delays, Billy Martin used to let Guidry play. When he left the Yankees, the drum set stayed.

Perhaps I owe a debt of gratitude to Guidry, because when I joined the Yankees, the tradition continued: Joe Torre would let Paul O'Neil (who is a pretty good drummer, if I may say so) and me jam in that same room. It was perhaps more for fun and to relax, but the two of us could do a mean version of Wilson Pickett's "Mustang Sally." I kept a guitar amp in the room, and during rain delays or after batting practices, Paul and I would jam to everything–the blues, Mellencamp, the Stones–you name it. Whenever Derek Jeter would turn on MTV to watch music videos in the clubhouse lounge, I'd try to play along on my guitar and learn every song.

When the Yankees were home, I'd go and hear as much live jazz in New York City as possible–Mike Stern at the Iridium, or Chick Corea's Electric Band with Eric Marienthal (saxophone), Chick Corea (keyboard), Frank Gambale (guitar), Victor Wooten (bass), and Dave Weckl (drums). David Wells and Paul O'Neil introduced me to Richie Sambora (of Bon Jovi), Bruce Springsteen (who signed my Fender Telecaster), Paul McCartney, Billy Joel, Creed, and others. One of the perks of being a New York Yankee was that you regularly got to meet artists like these–but since I was also a musician, the opportunity to hang with these legends was all the more inspiring.

While traveling with the Yankees, my guitar would travel too. On our plane, there were "unofficial" assigned seats, and mine was in the back of the plane behind Derek Jeter's. While Derek was listening to music on his headphones or trying to sleep, I'd always be practicing my guitar (or until Derek whacked the back of his seat enough times to get my attention, complaining that I was keeping him from getting some much needed rest).

Different rules applied back then aboard a Yankees charter flight–as opposed to flying commercial. Want to play your guitar during takeoffs? Sure–as long as you had your seat belt buckled. During landings and taxiing? Usually not a problem. The downside was that I ended up feeling like a flying lounge musician in the back of the plane, taking requests–Van Halen, Clapton, etc. Jeter had eclectic tastes–everything from R&B, Lionel Ritchie, etc.–and he'd try mumbling along with the vocals as I played. It was pure fun–and I got a lot of practice time in too.

I always looked forward to playing against the Angels in Anaheim–for the acoustics. There were these intertwining, interconnecting series of tunnels that led from the clubhouses to the main concourses and exits. The acoustics and natural reverb were amazing. I'd take a chair, go into one of the tunnels, and practice. While on the road with the Yankees, the first thing I'd do when I walked into a clubhouse or room was to clap my hands to test the acoustics.

During free evenings while on the road with the Yankees, I'd seek out live music wherever and whenever I could. One time I took my friend and teammate Tino Martinez to hear Sting play in concert after an afternoon game in Kansas City–Lyle Lovett was the opening act–and Sting and his band were amazing. I also remember hearing bands such as Def Leppard, White Snake, and Night Ranger (the guitarist Joel Hoekstra from Night Ranger is amazing). When I was out in Los Angeles, hearing guitarist Scott Henderson at the Baked Potato was a highlight as well. All these artists inspired me, and fueled my desire to excel on the field the next game.

It could be said that there are only two types of people that can fill Yankee Stadium: ballplayers and musicians (the Pope notwithstanding). The Beatles made Shea Stadium their first stop on their 1965 USA tour, and from the recordings I've heard of that concert, the fans were screaming so loud it sounded like a two-hour grand slam. I've always felt that there was this connection—a spirit and disposition—that great musicians and ballplayers shared.

I once stood in center field with Paul Simon, about a month after Joe DiMaggio's passing, and Paul asked me what it felt like to stand in one of the most majestic ballparks on the planet. Without thinking, I replied, "It feels like the Grand Canyon." And it does. Standing at the edge of the Grand Canyon, you're filled with wonderment. Center field at the old Yankee Stadium was no different. It occurred to me more than once while out in center—waiting for the pitcher's delivery—that I was on hallowed ground, waiting in anticipation the same way that Mickey Mantle, Joe DiMaggio, and Earle Combs once did standing in that very same patch of grass. As a musician, it's the same feeling standing on the stage of Carnegie Hall before a concert—or at Abbey Road before a recording session. They are all magical, mystical spaces—and you can't help but realize that you're part of a lineage—a tradition—of great musicians and ballplayers that preceded you.

Ken Burns, in his PBS documentary on baseball, described the sport as being comprised of "art and mystery." So is music. Everything about being a professional musician and a pro ballplayer is in pursuit of one thing—artistic perfection—that one fleeting, epiphanic moment. Baseball is a game of mental alchemy, and so is music—both can be reduced to mathematical combinations, statistics, and analysis—yet there is the uncertainty and mystery of what will be. As a Yankee, I couldn't wait to get to the outcome of the game—to find out if I would be the hero or the goat that day. I have the same feeling before every concert.

Baseball and music share other parallels too. Teams go on the road to play a series—rock bands go on the road to play a tour. A concert is a game, a song an inning, a musical phrase an at bat, and a single note played on a musical instrument is a swing of the bat (and of course—a swing and a miss equals a missed note—but more about that later).

I've often been asked how baseball has influenced my

life in music. I think it was actually the other way around: music influenced how I played baseball. The game, after all, is entirely built on rhythm, an essential element of music. Great players have an intuitive sense of rhythm, the effect of which is great timing. Every at bat and every play has its own rhythm to it, and music is the undercurrent. From Miles Davis one can learn that, no matter what selection of notes you have to play, they don't mean a thing if they're not played in precisely the right space, time, and with the appropriate level of nuance. The same is true of baseball.

My background in music gave me something else that greatly affected my ability on the field: resilience and determination to accomplish the task at hand. That resilience came from my weekly guitar lessons. I'd come home from school on Thursdays, finish my homework, and then run off to my guitar lesson followed by baseball practice. I never saw practicing guitar as a chore–but it was the guitar that made me realize that, even though I was young, I had control over my life.

If I was resilient and determined in my practicing, I would progress and be able to play the music I really wanted to play. I also learned that I could easily transfer the discipline and focus of practicing my guitar to sports–or anything else. When you're seven years old and realize that the musical instrument you're holding in your hands empowers you to do whatever you want in life, it's a breakthrough moment. Consequently, my parents never had to tell me to practice–nor did they ever have to tell me to put my baseball uniform on either.

Young aspiring musicians spend an inordinate amount of time–thousands of hours–in solitude honing their craft. The art of practicing–sitting alone in a room with nothing else but your instrument and the music on the page–is a very humbling experience. Young musicians aspiring to a career on the concert stage are called upon very early in life to sacrifice hours a day in the pursuit of perfection. As a young musician growing up in Puerto Rico, I learned from my parents the need for this level of resilience and determination if I was going to be successful. Transferring these qualities from music to baseball was invaluable in my development as a ballplayer. I've learned much from music and applied those very same musical concepts to baseball.

At times, the game became a dance–and when I was rhythmically in sync with that dance, it was magic. The pitch, the swing, and the contact with the ball were all part of a tango with an odd-metered musical undertone. The rhythm of a pitcher going into his windup and throwing the ball is a form of music in and of itself. As a hitter, rocking back and forth and timing the pitcher was a musically intuitive process for me–like music without a time signature. The feeling I got from hitting the ball on the sweet spot of the bat and seeing it fly out of the park is remarkably similar to the feeling I derive from improvising a well-executed musical line on my guitar during a concert. Both feel as if they were composed for that singular moment, and although each lasts but for a few fleeting seconds, the experience is remarkably similar, profound, and inspiring.

When I played for the Yankees, I'd be acutely aware of the rhythms of the game–when I was at bat, naturally–but also when I played in the outfield. Take for example a double play, where rhythm is usually synchronized around three players. In a well-executed double play, the players have to anticipate each other's movements and rhythms, just like great jazz musicians do. In my mind, a great double play is no different than a great all-star rhythm section–Count Basie on piano, Walter Page on bass, and Philly Jo Jones on drums–performing perfectly in sync with a groove unlike no other. Every great double play has a great jazz rhythm section as its soundtrack.

Breathing is another element I brought from music to the game. Music is about breathing–whether you're playing a trumpet or a guitar–as every phrase begins with a musical breath. Breathing in music is as much artistry as it is a necessity for singers, but breathing has an important role in baseball as well.

In clutch situations, bottom of the ninth with two men out and the game hanging in the balance with your next swing, breathing can have an extraordinary influence on your game. It helps you slow things down, step back, stay organized, and keeps you in control of your approach. It renders stillness and calm. Focused breathing has also helped me with other aspects of the game–from endurance and concentration to pacing and timing. It's impossible to have a relaxed swing if you're breathing isn't relaxed as well.

Being flexible musically–learning as much as I could about all styles of music and learning to improvise–enabled me to be a more flexible ballplayer. I was probably 70 percent a reactionary hitter, and music is all about how you react–and act–in key situations. In addition to playing music, I compose music too. Music composition is akin to managing a group of notes and rhythms that, when ordered in a special way, creates something magical, not unlike how a manager like Joe Torre or a pitcher like Andy Pettitte "compose" a game plan.

It wasn't until I left baseball that I began to realize how much my music and my guitar meant to me during my career with the Yankees. I used it for everything–to relax before a big game, to keep me focused during rain delays, to vent when things weren't going well, and to channel my energies off the field in a positive, nonverbal way. It kept me sane during difficult times and allowed me to express joy during the good ones. Baseball made me a better musician while music made me a better ballplayer. Thus, it's no wonder to me that great musicians and ballplayers have held one another in great admiration. The skill set required to be a great musician is very similar to what's required to play major league ball at a high level.

Music and baseball share a connection unlike any other between two disciplines within sports and the arts. Ironically, despite my musical background, I was one of the few players that purposely didn't want any music played when I got up at the plate. I didn't really need it. The purest, most musical sounds of baseball are those of the spectators–of umpires making calls, coaches and players shouting, of parents yelling as their kid gets a hit–and nothing else. For me, the sounds of the game are inherently musical, and there are times backstage when I hear the crowd in the concert hall and, despite holding a guitar in my hands and not a bat–it's all the same. I know I'm on deck. In a few minutes, I'll have a two-hour at bat and I'm going to cherish every minute of it.

# 4
# The Matrix Moment

## Achieving peak performance
## on the field or onstage

*I always get very calm with baseball.*
–PAUL SIMON

Let me put you in my shoes for a moment: imagine what it feels like to be at bat at Yankee Stadium–bottom of the ninth, you're down three runs, the bases are loaded, and you're facing an 0–2 count. Notch it up a bit–perhaps it's the American League Championship Series and this is the deciding Game 7. The crowd of 50,000-plus is pounding the concrete, screaming in a collective, deafening roar. You can't hear yourself think, and yet the entire weight of the stadium–and perhaps the entire New York Yankees season–hangs on your next swing.

Maybe the batter isn't me–maybe the batter is none other than Paul Simon, who's standing offstage right, about to walk on. Except it's not a 50,000-seat stadium–it's Central Park in New York City, and there are now 500,000 screaming fans waiting in anticipation. HBO is there to film it, along with a recording crew that will release the live album. Is your guitar tuned? How's your voice? Are you nervous yet?

For many folks, the thought of being in this moment–at bat in an intense pressure situation, or about to take the mike in front of 500,000 people–would be a terrifying experience. You'd expect to be nervous, have butterflies in your stomach, feel your knees shaking, etc. For some, panic would set in. All these reactions are totally normal and expected, given the gravity of the moment. All of us, including professional ballplayers and musicians, have experienced nervousness at some time or another.

But imagine another scenario in which all these feelings of insecurity, dread, and nervousness are squashed. Imagine that instead of these feelings, you feel calm, focused, and totally in control. Imagine that you feel so totally locked in that there is nothing standing between you and achieving something extraordinary.

Imagine owning the moment.

You can tell when a player owns the moment–there's almost this precognition among the fans or the audience that a player is going to make something happen. There's no doubt about it. Certain ballplayers and artists have "the aura"–a level of confidence that is almost mythical.

Take David "Big Papi" Ortiz for instance, when he was in his prime with the Boston Red Sox. He'd be facing an 0–2 count and the pitcher was in control (or so he thought)–then Big Papi would call time and step back–just like the mythical, mighty Casey. He'd spit on his gloves, rub his hands together, take the bat–and then he'd get that look in his eyes–and everyone knew it was the "oh no" moment. Everyone–from the players to the fans–knew he was going to make something happen. It wasn't, "Is he gonna do it?" It was, "He's gonna do it!" He owned the moment.

There are musicians like this as well. When Bono takes the mike, Clapton picks up the guitar, or Itzhak Perlman picks up his violin–before they sing or play–you just know they're going to make something special happen. They own the moment too. There's an aura around them–a level of calm confidence. Hopefully, in your career as a musician or a ballplayer, you will experience this moment, and when it happens, it will be a revelation to you. You are in the zone.

Being "in the zone" is a rarified place where your preparation and experience, coupled with your intuition, bring you to a higher realm: your body is relaxed but working at peak efficiency–your mind is clear, calm, and focused–and despite a roaring crowd in their seats, you are totally in a Zen-like state of command. You're so focused and locked in that time seems to slow down. Rather than nerves, you feel like that moment in the film *The Matrix* where Keanu

Reaves first discovers that he has total mastery over time and space—and total mastery over the moment. It is an extraordinary place to be in—the pressure of the moment and the roar of the crowd only bring you further into the zone and that "Matrix Moment" where you are in complete control.

One of my earliest professional experiences of being "in the zone" was back in 1996—specifically, a windy New York night on October 9. It was Game 1 of the American League Championship Series against the Baltimore Orioles. Older Yankees fans will remember that this was back in the day when a twenty-two-year-old Derek Jeter batted ninth, Andy Pettitte was twenty-four years old, and the Yankees were a team of virtual unknowns. In fact, Bob Costas, the TV announcer for the game, quipped, "This Yankee team is unlike the era of Ruth, Gehrig, DiMaggio, Jackson, etc. This team has no superstar." He was right. We were unknown. We had lost the division series the year before against the Seattle Mariners. A year later, we were back in the playoffs—this time advancing to the ALCS against the legendary Cal Ripkin and the Baltimore Orioles. We were excited as a team—we had won the division series against Texas, losing the first game, 6–2, but sweeping them in the next three.

The wind was blowing like crazy on this October night—a routine fly ball in the first inning by Tim Raines was lost by the Orioles' left fielder, and due to Raines's hustling, he made it to second. It was a classic example of how great players never assume anything—he ran so hard on that fly ball that, when the ball was dropped, he was able to turn it into a double.

The game was emotionally charged and controversial too—the home plate umpire was calling an unusually wide strike zone, with pitchers getting strike calls way off of the plate, which made it frustrating for us as hitters. This, however, is part of the game, and it requires you to adjust accordingly. Manager Joe Torre would remind us that the other team would face the same strike zone, so it works both ways.

The most controversial moment came with the Yankees trailing the Baltimore Orioles, 4–3, in the eighth inning. In what would be called the infamous "Jeffrey Maier" home run (not to mention Jeter's first postseason home run), Jeter hit a fly ball to deep right field. Tony Tarasco jumped up against the wall to catch it just as twelve-year-old Jeffrey Maier, a young fan in the first row seats, reached over the wall and caught the ball, pulling it back into the stands. Despite Tarasco's protest, the umpires ruled the ball a home run. The home run tied the game, and kept the Yankees in business, but the score remained tied into extra innings. Now fast-forward to the eleventh inning.

In the top of the eleventh, I'm out in center field—and in between pitches, I'm envisioning the variables I'll face in the bottom half of the inning. If the Orioles don't score, I'm going to be leading off the bottom of the eleventh inning with the score tied. What do I want this at bat to look like? What do I want to create? I'm operating simultaneously now in the present and the future—focusing on defense when Mariano Rivera has the ball and then switching to the bottom of the eleventh and envisioning this crucial at bat.

Back and forth, it went like this for the top of the eleventh. I'm imagining all the possible scenarios in which I could potentially find myself when I approach the plate. I wasn't imagining hitting the ball out of the park. I just knew I needed to make something happen—to have a good at bat, get on base—and I knew that as long as I could get on base, I could make something happen.

There was something else I focused on at this moment: for the first time in the game, I would be batting from my stronger side—the right side.

Mariano Rivera got us out of the inning, and I ran off the field back to the dugout. I became hyper-focused at this point—totally blocking out the roar of the crowd and the pressure of the moment—and I felt calm and relaxed—the exact opposite of what you would normally expect to feel in this high-pressure moment.

When I got to the plate, the only two people in the ballpark in my mind were Orioles closer Randy Myers and me. At that moment, we could easily have been two guys playing ball in an Iowa cornfield. The crowd had disappeared, the pressure and nerves were gone, and everything started to slow down. I was amped up, ready to go—with a "Bring it on!" mentality. I'm totally in the present—in "the now".

My eyes lock on to every movement of Randy Myers—and his first pitch I let go by. It's a ball.

I now make a crucial decision. I'm up, 1–0, and if the next pitch is a strike, I'm going to let it go by as well. This next pitch is for the team—the more pitches they can see from Myers, the better—so I'm giving it up, and it's likely going to be a strike.

And Myers does exactly what my intuition tells me—he throws a strike, and I take it.

It's at this point where my mind and body are totally in sync. I'm feeling confident, I'm batting from my strong side, and I know that this next pitch could likely be "the moment" for me. I know that I've worked hard to get here—the years of practice, of daily routines and drills, and that my teammates have all worked hard too in order to give me this moment. This at bat is a gift.

In this hyper-focused state, I feel confident and blessed. It's a moment every young kid (myself included) dreams of being in—postseason, extra innings, the game hanging in the balance with your next swing. I have no control over the outcome of this game, but I do have control over my approach to this at bat, which I'd envisioned in my mind in the outfield during the top half of the inning.

When the next pitch comes on a 1-1 count, I experience a surreal moment. Time slows down so much that I'm able to stop, put down my bat, grab a camera, and take a picture of the ball leaving Myers's hand. I can see the speed of the ball and its location. It's a hanging breaking ball. And it's going to be up and away.

The ball seems huge—like a beach ball. Time had slowed to the point where I could actually take and process this mental snapshot, and I knew in this instant that I had locked into Myers's timing. There was no way I could miss it.

The ball is indeed a breaking ball up and away. I swing— "Crush it" is more how it feels—and because the ball hangs somewhat—I pull it—and the ball rockets off into left field.

At this moment, I can't quite comprehend what's happening. In some ways, the moment reminds me of my first Little League game–I was seven years old and the local police athletic association in my town organized games for us kids. I knew nothing about the rules of baseball–and had no interest in the sport, but my dad thought it would be a good idea for my brother, Hiram, and I to get out of the house and get some exercise, so off we went to the ball field. I didn't want to play, so I hung out by the bench playing in the sand, oblivious to anything happening on the field. After an hour or so, the coach yelled for me to get up and bat. Reluctantly, I got up, swung at the ball–and then something strange happened: everybody started walking off the field. The game was over. I ran up to the coach, who was walking away, and asked, "What happened? Why is the game over? Did I do something wrong?" The coach explained that the game was tied with runners on base, and I had hit a line drive that had driven home the winning run in the bottom of the last inning. I was a bit disappointed, though–my first baseball game, and it was over before I even knew what was going on.

Back at Yankee Stadium, I start to allow the crowd in–I can hear the noise, and I see the ball sail into the left field stands. The game is over–just like my first Little League game–and we had won Game 1.

When I watched the video of this game with Bob and Dave for the first time recently–after fourteen years–I also realized how being in the zone at this moment gave me the ability to (and this is important) temper the moment. Yes, it was a walk-off home run in the playoffs that won the game for the Yankees–but it was only Game 1. I know that great players never truly let the highs and lows of the game affect them too much, and as a young Yankee center fielder, I was trying to be like those great players who came before me. If you let the highs in too much, you're bound to let the lows in too much as well. Better to keep yourself focused and even-keeled.

This at bat in Game 1 of the 1996 ALCS is as close as I can describe, in words, to what being "in the zone" means. I have been blessed by many other moments as well. The only thing that compares to this, outside of baseball, has been music. There have been times while practicing my guitar, where I'm improvising over a chord progression, and I'll be focusing totally on the creative aspect of my music, blocking out any critical thoughts. I cease to be a guitarist at this moment and begin to enter the realm of the artist. In other words, there's a "tabula rasa" before me–a blank canvas–much like that at bat in 1996–and I am in the zone.

I'll record myself during these "in the zone" sessions–that's what they are–practice sessions designed to get me focused and in the zone, so that I'm no longer practicing but creating. What amazes me is that, when I listen back to the tape, I'll notice sometimes that I'm able to create something entirely different, new–something that my analytical left brain couldn't imagine. I'll remark, "Hey, that was cool–I wonder how I got to the point of playing *that!*" Sometimes, I don't even remember what I did. I've had many at bats like this, where I was in a place of creativity and artistry that so enveloped my consciousness that I can't remember what happened–I have to watch the replay.

I've had these uncommon experiences onstage too–performing with my band. Most recently, I did a concert at the Lafayette Theater in Suffern, New York, and I remember feeling very much "in the zone." The crowd was cheering, and I was improvising a solo, when suddenly I'm transported to a place where I'm focused, relaxed, and time slows down. It was an amazing experience.

When I'm in the zone, it doesn't matter how difficult the passage is or how fast the tune. When I listened to the tape from the performance, I was somewhat taken aback by what happened onstage that night. And many times, I can't recall it having happened until I listen to the playback. In this way, musicians and ballplayers share this uncommon place–this zone where creativity and artistry live. The feeling I have in this rarified place is the same regardless of whether I'm holding a guitar or a holding a bat, and it's one of the most profound parallels between music and baseball. The guitar, the bat, the glove–they all simply become extensions of your creative voice. Everything feels light. Everything feels relaxed.

When you're in the zone, you're concentrating so fully that you're not affected by the small details–how many balls or strikes, whether you missed a note or not, whether you struck out during your last at bat. Nothing distracts you (whether it's 10,000 fans cheering you on while performing onstage, or 37,000 angry Red Sox fans cheering for your demise at Fenway). It is a realm free of criticism. It's transcendent, spiritual in nature, and one of the greatest gifts that can be bestowed on any athlete or artist.

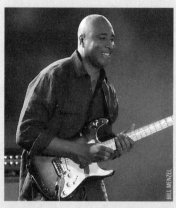

# BIOLOGY TEST

by Bernie Williams

This state of being relaxed, focused, and calm is what Don Greene (in the sidebar to the chapter "Batting Practice") calls the "alpha state." In the alpha state, your brainwaves actually slow down. When you first wake up in the morning–relaxed and calm–you're in the alpha state. As you awake and start your day, your brainwaves speed up, and you're in the "beta state."

The first time I experienced the alpha state–where I actually made it happen–was at my performing-arts high school in Puerto Rico. There was a biology exam, and a friend of mine was telling me about the "alpha" and "beta" states of consciousness. So I tried an experiment: I didn't study for the exam. I had taken good notes during class, but I wanted to test and see if I could put myself into a stressful, pressured situation–yet remain relaxed and focused. When I took the exam, I was "in the zone," just like the at bat in the bottom of the eleventh in Game 1 of the 1996 ALCS.

In both instances, I was definitely in an alpha state. And the strange thing is, all the knowledge and skill I had learned in the beta state while taking notes in class poured into my alpha state while taking the exam. It was an amazing experience–and I ended up with the highest mark in the school for that exam. It proved to me that there was another way to achieve peak performance–not through working less hard–but working just as hard, correctly! If you can put yourself in an alpha state during a peak-performance situation, it's akin to fully opening the faucet and unlocking the power of your mind and the skill and talent that is within you.

# THE MATRIX MOMENT

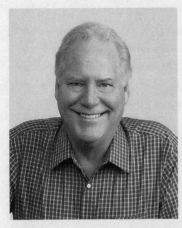

## ANALYZING "THE MATRIX MOMENT"

by Don Greene, Ph.D., sports and music psychologist

What Bernie Williams experienced in that eleventh-inning bat in Game 1 of the 1996 ALCS can be described through science and flow psychology. It's the result of being in the alpha state (which I discuss in detail at the end of the "Batting Practice" chapter).

In the flow state, the ego falls away. Time distorts. Every thought, action, and movement follows fluidly from the previous one, like playing jazz. Your whole being is involved, and you're using your skills to the utmost. Flow could be thought of as a state where focused attention, strong motivation, and a challenging situation intersect, resulting in a productive harmony.

Flow is the mental state of a person engaged in a chosen activity, immersed in a feeling of energized focus and full involvement. Flow is completely focused motivation, a single-minded absorption into a physical event. In flow, the emotions are not just contained, but are positive, energized, and channeled into the task at hand. The hallmark of flow is a feeling of spontaneous joy while performing a challenging activity at the peak of one's abilities.

There are a number of conditions that are essential in order for performers and competitors to experience the flow state. They must begin the activity with clear overall goals, with many intermediate checkpoints along the way. In a chess game, each player wants to win, but they need to know, with every move, if they're getting closer to winning or losing. Musicians and athletes need immediate and continuing feedback about how they're sounding or playing. If they hit a wrong note or make an error, they need to know, so they can immediately correct the mistake. Accurate feedback is essential to keeping on track.

In flow states, there is a balance between the level or difficulty of the challenge and the participant's ability and skill level to meet that challenge. When activities are too easy, not requiring full involvement or attention, people get bored and are easily distracted. If the activities are way beyond people's ability or skill level, they get intimidated, anxious, defensive, frustrated, and often give up—or at the very least—they don't enjoy the experience. And that's another point. These activities are also to be enjoyed for their own sake, for the pure pleasure of experiencing them.

When people are engaged in challenging activities that require a high degree of concentration, they're able to get beyond the normal experience of everyday consciousness, with life's daily frustrations, worries, and doubts. If they're performing live music or playing in a game, they can't be thinking about normal stuff, or they'll miss a note or make an error. They can't afford to let their minds wander, like they can while walking down the supermarket aisle.

Professional musicians and outstanding baseball players understand the difference between what happens in normal, everyday circumstances and highly challenging situations, like performing live in front of thousands of fans. Routine activities, like opening the mail or shopping for food, don't require—and hence don't get—our undivided attention. So we get in the habit of splitting our attention between several things that we're able to do at the same time, like shopping while talking on a cell phone and making plans for the weekend.

But in highly challenging situations, like performing live solos or needing to get a hit, demand nothing less than total attention. Other less critical concerns—like what we're going to do on the weekend—quickly disappear. In the flow state, the attention that is usually split between things is merged into a single, highly concentrated beam of focused consciousness. Performers and athletes who are in flow are much more focused, efficient in their actions, and tend to produce successful outcomes.

Even in extremely challenging situations, when done in flow, there is a feeling of being in control of your experience and actions. But this is not the feeling of being in complete control of the situation; otherwise, the activity wouldn't be challenging enough for your level of skills or abilities. In the flow state, you are always on an edge. It is an edge where control is possible, but not guaranteed. You can fall off the edge if you lose your focus or don't use your skills to their full potential. That's what makes it exciting and demanding.

Musicians' and athletes' sense of time is distorted or transformed when they're in flow. When totally absorbed in an extended riff or extra-innings game, time can seem to pass very quickly. Other times, moments can seem to slow down or even stop. The perception of time adapts to the external events and how you experience them when you're in flow.

When musicians and athletes are engaged in activities that challenge their highest abilities, there is a lack of self-consciousness, a loss of ego. In flow, you don't about what other people may think of you and your performance. There is a feeling of transcendence, because you're forced to forget about yourself—and how you're thought of—as you get beyond the ego.

In flow, there is a merging of effortless action and awareness. People become completely absorbed in the activity and what they're doing. The focus of their awareness is narrowed down to the task at hand and nothing else. Then there is a required surrendering, or "letting go," to the experience or activity. You need to be able to let it go.

People with certain personality traits are better able to achieve flow states. These traits include open-mindedness, persistence, and a preference for high-action situations demanding high skills and total attention—which cause them to enter into flow, become highly alert, and transcend ordinary consciousness. Individuals with these traits are said to have an "autotelic personality."

The autotelic personality has five characteristics, known as the "five Cs." The first is *clarity*: setting clear goals and knowing what you want to accomplish; and clarity of feedback, to know how you're doing on a moment-to-moment basis until the goal is achieved. The second is the ability to *center*—to focus your full attention on what you're doing in the here and now.

The third characteristic is *choice*—knowing that you have chosen to do this activity. You're not being forced; you want to do it. Hopefully, you also really enjoy it. The fourth is the ability to *commit* yourself fully to what you're doing and care deeply about how you're doing it. The fifth characteristic of an auto-telic personality is continually upping the *challenge* after mastering a certain level, which involves the progressive raising of one's abilities and skill level.

The flow state has a strong correlation with the further development of one's skills. When musicians and athletes are in flow, they are working to master their chosen activity. To experience the flow state, you must seek increasingly greater challenges. Attempting new and difficult challenges stretches and expands your skills and abilities, including more frequent experiences of flow. You emerge from such experiences with feelings of competence and efficacy, and an even higher motivation to perform well.

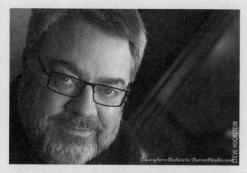

## JAZZ BALL

. . . . . . . . . . . . . . . . . . . . . . . . . . . . . . . . . . . . . .

by Todd Coolman, Grammy-
winning jazz bassist with
Horace Silver, Gerry Mulligan,
Stan Getz, and James Moody,
among many others

. . . . . . . . . . . . . . . . . . . . . . . . . . . . . . . . . . . . . .

Both jazz and baseball involve ever-changing, moment-to-moment circumstances that require the participant to analyze, conceptualize, adapt, adjust to, and ultimately improvise within. Both the jazz musician and baseball player are dealing with a finite array of known data and methodology, and both must arrange these tools in a fashion that allows for the most appropriate implementation at that moment.

Both the jazz musician and baseball player must be conversant in a nomenclature of sorts, and must know something about the mindset and varied abilities and sensibilities of their teammates. Both must work within a flow and must be able, in turn, to go with the flow as it continually redirects itself. For the pitcher and catcher, for instance, it can be a pitch-by-pitch occurrence. Similarly, jazz music can change on the instant of one particular beat, chord, or melody. For the jazz musician, this can also be a "pitch-by-pitch" scenario.

Ultimately, the most successful jazz musicians and baseball players are not necessarily the most talented, but are always the best prepared, consistent, and aware of the "big picture" of the game. Both must be simultaneously in the moment, and also aware of the architecture of the entire game, from the first pitch or beat until the last. They must be in a constant state of readiness for both the expected and unexpected.

# MO' MATRIX: FLOW AND PEAK PERFORMANCE

by Don Greene

To review, the characteristics of flow are: (1) the skill level matching the challenge of the task; (2) the merging of action and awareness; (3) clearly defined goals; (4) immediate and continuous feedback; (5) total concentration on the task at hand; (6) letting go; (7) the loss of self-consciousness; and (8) the perceived transformation of time.

A peak performance is a temporary episode of superior functioning, characterized by exceptional playing, as in athletic and artistic contexts. An event becomes a peak performance when the superior action is accompanied by a sharp focus and clear intent, and a strong sense of self in process, leading to a feeling of self-validation and fulfillment.

The qualities of peak performances are a loss of fear, no thinking of performance, full focus of attention, total immersion and absorption in the chosen activity, and the feeling of being godlike (in control). These qualities are also accompanied by the perception of separate things as being integrated, unified, and whole–with time-space disorientation, a feeling of awe, wonder, and appreciation following the self-transcendent experience.

Peak performances also require being physically and mentally prepared, feeling confident and optimistic, focused in the present, with highly energized, extraordinary awareness, and being in a cocoon of concentration. There are also feelings of positive expectation of success, acting completely in the moment, being spontaneous with a sense of possessing extraordinary power, being completely absorbed and immersed in the activity, and experiencing feelings of total joy and ecstasy.

The characteristics shared by both peak performances and flow states are: total absorption and involvement in the chosen activity, a sense of joy, valuing the temporary experience, spontaneity and freedom, the awareness of exceptional power, altered perceptions of time, and a sense of connectedness, unity, and harmony.

# 5
# The Intuitive Artist

Understanding musical and
athletic intuition

*Improvised music involves a lot of intuition*
*and I like developing intuition.*
–FRED FRITH

*The creative is the place where no one else has ever*
*been. You have to leave the city of your comfort and go*
*into the wilderness of your intuition.*
–ALAN ALDA

There is nothing more profound in sports than watching an amazing play unfold before you on the field. Great players, having crystallized their approach and fundamentals to such a point where they cease to become athletes, rise to a level of artistry that transcends the sport itself and enters a realm that can only be described as art in motion.

Michael Jordan and Wayne Gretzky are two such examples. To describe Jordan and Gretzky simply as amazing athletes doesn't do them justice. At their peaks, each had risen above athleticism, moving to a realm where artists create and inspire. Great musicians are like that too–watching guitarist Jimmy Page or violinist Itzhak Perlman perform is a lot like watching Michael Jordan in action. They've mastered their craft at such a high level that they dominate and create an entirely new realm for all to aspire to. These artists are few and far between–the number of true artists in any one field, despite the hundreds of exceptional ones, is but a handful.

What is it about artists like Michael Jordan or Itzhak Perlman that place them in this rarified air of excelling beyond our imagination? There are three prerequisites: (1) total mastery of their craft, (2) depth and quality of experience, and–the most elusive–(3) an exceptionally heightened level of intuition that draws on the first two. Intuition is different from instinct, and many players confuse the terms. Instinct is purely physical and hereditary–a pitcher ducks when a line drive is hit at his head–that's instinct. Intuition, on the other hand, is a brain function. Having the knowledge, coupled with a level of cognition, in the absence of rational thought is intuition. And unlike instinct, intuition can be refined and developed.

Many great players rise to the level of having a firm grasp on mastery and experience, and their level of intuition might be exceptional, but it is only those rare few that have a level of uncanny intuition that places them above all others. Conversely, there are some great players who have this heightened level of intuition–what one might call "an elasticity of thinking"–yet they don't possess the mastery and/or experience. It's one of the facets of major league baseball that make it so compelling–you can be successful with perhaps just one or two of these three traits. But it is only the rare few–the artists of the game–that have mastery over all three.

Like grandmaster chess players, these artists can see the big picture and intuitively think ahead four or five moves, whereas a decent chess player can only see one or two moves forward. My colleague Roberto Alomar, who was also from Puerto Rico, had this unique ability. Perhaps the greatest second baseman to ever play the game, Roberto had this ability on occasion to intuitively throw behind the runner trying to score from first on a ball to the gap (which is something you're not taught to do) and get him out. His intuition would compel him to do this, and more times than not, he would get the runner out. The same ability and experience in the hands of another second baseman would result in disaster. But not Alomar!

This level of intuition can only come about from having a tremendous amount of experience behind you, coupled with complete mastery of the game. There is a certain level of unreasonable, unbridled confidence that great artists have in committing to this type of play at this level. There is total commitment in executing a play like Alomar used to make. There is absolutely no second-guessing ("Should I throw behind the runner?"). The decision is made intuitively. It can't be learned and it can't be taught. It can, however, be developed.

A good place to develop intuition is on first base when you're deciding whether to steal or not. You're studying the pitcher, your body feeds your brain important information, and without being totally 100 percent conscious of the moment, your mind and body commit and you're off to second base. There is no hesitation in this process and no second-guessing yourself either. At the moment that your mind and body commit to the decision, you execute fully. Great artists make these decisions unaware or unaffected by the outcome–"What if I get caught stealing?" These thoughts of failure simply don't enter their minds.

In order for these moments of brilliance to happen, your body has to be operating at its peak–in baseball, you have to be feeling particularly strong physically–and your mind has to be at a heightened level of awareness that can identify opportunities and react–and act–accordingly. This type of awareness and focus makes you able to instantly evaluate, interpret, and react–sometimes thinking totally outside the box–or the diamond.

Here's a classic example of a player who has honed his fundamentals and basics to such a high level that, when put into practice, the result is a work of art. The example has simply been called, "The Moment."

It was the seventh inning in Game 3 of the 2001 American League Division Series, and Yankees starter Mike Mussina was pitching like an ace, having allowed just a pair of hits and no runs in a pitcher's duel with A's left-hander Barry Zito. The Yankees were leading, 1–0, on a Jorge Posada home run.

With Mussina on the mound with two outs, and Jeremy Giambi leading off first, Terrence Long hits a ground ball inside the first-base line, just past the reach of Yankees first baseman, Tino Martinez. The ball bounces down the right-field line as Giambi rounds second, and is being told to keep going by the third-base coach, Ron Washington. The Yankees' right fielder, Shane Spencer, runs toward the corner, hoping to reach the ball before it hits the wall while Alfonso Soriano, playing second base, sprints into short right field to get in position for the cutoff, and Martinez positions himself near the first-base bag, backing up Soriano. Everyone is exactly where they need to be. Except, something goes awry.

Derek Jeter is, of course, in his proper place—near the pitcher's mound, where he's in a position to either cut off a throw to third base, move to back up the two relay players, or cover second base in the event of a throw to nail Long at second. Out in right field, Spencer grabs the ball, whirls, and fires toward home plate as Giambi rounds third. Scott Brosius later commented, "He'd be out by ten feet if we make a good relay." But that's not what happened. Spencer's strong throw not only sails over Soriano's head, but also over Martinez's.

It's at this point that everyone realizes Giambi is going to score, the game will be tied, and the A's—who won the first two games of the best-of-five series—could wrap it up with another run. Everyone knows that Giambi is gonna score and there is nothing to be done—everyone except the artist at shortstop, Derek Jeter.

If you were watching the game on TV, what happened next can only be described as impossible and jaw dropping. With the television camera zooming in on the area between first base and home plate, Jeter appears out of nowhere, running across the screen, swooping in from the middle of the infield running toward the first-base line. The first thought as you see him totally out of position and in the middle of the television screen is, "What is he doing there?" It looked like a fan running across the infield (albeit a fan in a Yankees uniform). Jeter runs to the first baseline, scoops up the ball with two hands on a bounce in foul territory and—still in motion— laterally flips the ball backhanded twenty feet to Posada, much like a quarterback who pitches the football in an option play. It's a perfect pass to Posada, who only needs to reach back and tag Giambi. Inning over.

The Oakland players are aghast, speechless. The crowd is still trying to process what just happened. The announcers are trying to comprehend it too, and multiple replays are shown. "What was he even doing in that spot?" Johnny Damon later cried, to which Terrence Long added, "He had no business there whatsoever!" The A's manager, Art Howe, in a postgame interview, put it best: "I don't have a clue as to how or why he was even involved in that play. Shows what kind of player he is."

What does this example tell us? Teams don't ordinarily practice plays to figure out where they put a third relay player. If a ball is overthrown to both cutoff players, it's the catcher's job to get the ball. Had Jeter figured out this play in his mind ahead of time? He must have seen that Spencer's throw was going to go over Martinez's head and dashed in between Martinez at first and Posada at home. Had he practiced it? Well, it's unlikely that Jeter had an idea what he was going to do, nor did he have the time to think about it.

Like a great jazz musician, Jeter has mastered the mechanics and basics of baseball to a point that, when he's on the field, he is thoroughly prepared and in command of any situation, able to use his intuitive and creative right brain to make his body do what it needs to in order to turn routine into artistry. This can't be taught, but it can be acquired. The only path to this level of creativity, just as with a great jazz pianist, is through mastery of the basics and fundamentals, which allows your creative mind to improvise a work of art for just the right moment in space and time. And Jeter's play on that October day was nothing short of a masterwork of art.

That single play turned around the ALDS for the Yankees. We were down, 2–0, in the series, about to lose the third game, and the Yankees turned the entire series around on that one play, going on to win that day, as well as the next two games. There are a myriad of great diving, leaping catches and exceptionally well-turned double plays, but it is unlikely we'll ever see a play like this again.

# YOUR MUSICAL BRAIN ON BASEBALL

| LEFT BRAIN | RIGHT BRAIN |
| --- | --- |
| Words and Numbers | Sounds, Pictures, Sensations |
| Logic and Mathematics | Music and Art |
| Best for Practice | Best for Performing/Playing |
| Suboptimal Performance | Optimal and Peak Performance |
| Separation and Analysis | Synthesis and Intuition |
| Doubt and Self-Criticism | Confidence and Acceptance |
| Mental Noise and Scattered | Mental Quiet and Focused |
| Skepticism, Past and Future | Trusting, The Now |
| Staccato, Robotic | Flowing, Imaginative |
| Powerless Effort | Effortless Power |
| Judgment and Exclusion | Discernment and Inclusion |
| Absolute Time, Sequential | Relative Time, Simultaneous |
| Definitions, Facts | Interpretations, Meaning |
| Either/Or, This or That | Both and All |
| Rote and Tradition | New and Spontaneous |
| Thinking in Twos | Thinking in Threes or more |
| Pass/Fail and Black/White | Nuances, Subtleties, Gray Areas |

# BEHIND THE INTUITIVE ARTIST

by Don Greene

To understand the intuitive artistry of Derek Jeter's amazing play in Oakland back in 2001, we need to look at how "intuition" actually works. As Bernie said, intuition can be developed, but only if you know how to develop it. First, though, we need to understand how our brain functions.

The thinking part of the brain, or cerebral cortex, is divided into the left and right hemispheres. The left brain thinks in terms of words and numbers. The right brain perceives through images, sounds, and sensations.

Both the left and right hemispheres program the subconscious mind. The left brain programs the subconscious mind with words and numbers. The right brain uses pictures, sounds, and the tactile feeling of an experience.

The subconscious is by far the more powerful part of our minds. It's within the subconscious where our all-important confidence and self-beliefs reside. Although it's very powerful in producing results, the subconscious has some limitations worth noting.

The subconscious mind is very gullible. It will believe whatever the left brain tells it repeatedly and the right brain imagines. It cannot distinguish between reality and whatever is said over and over to oneself, what is vividly imagined. It believes anything it is programmed to, whether it's real or not.

The left brain tends to talk continually and incessantly. It's a noise machine. The subconscious listens and believes what it hears. It is very literal and doesn't have a sense of humor. Even if you think you're just joking about messing something up, your subconscious will follow the instruction very seriously and likely produce a mistake.

The subconscious mind has its own language that is somewhat foreign to our normal speech patters. It prefers pictures and functions according to its own rules. For example, it does not understand words like *won't* or *don't*, only what comes after them.

So consider what you're telling your subconscious to do if you say to yourself, "Don't miss this shot." It's much better to say, "Hit the shot." If you admit that something is "hard," it will soon prove to be so. The subconscious responds better to "challenging" than "hard" or "difficult."

The subconscious also interprets questions as statements. "Can I really do that?" is a statement that you don't think you can. Many elite performers are their own worst critics. Whether they realize it or not, those words have a serious impact on their subconscious minds and their confidence.

The conscious mind is continually programming the subconscious either toward success or failure, with more or less confidence. Self-confidence is never static: it is either rising or falling. The current level of one's self-belief is the direct result of their recent programming, either negatively or positively.

Negative programming includes doubts, worries, imagining failure, self-criticism, and making counter-productive interpretations about outside events. Positive programming includes supportive self-talk, imagining success, and self-serving interpretations about external circumstances.

When programmed with doubts, criticism, worries, imagined failure, and doomsday scenarios, confidence will fall. When programmed with positive thoughts, images of success, and positive interpretations, confidence will rise.

Unless it is unrealistic or arrogant, it is usually better to have more confidence than less. Since people tend to perform only at or below their level of self-belief, the goal is to continually raise one's confidence.

The goal is to convince your subconscious mind that you can do something. The threefold way to do that is through positive thoughts or affirmations, positive images or guided visualization, and right physical actions—like good practice habits.

# LESTER AND BILLIE

by Bernie, Dave, and Bob

Great musicians have extraordinary intuition. A guitarist like Pat Metheny, for instance, is able to respond appropriately and intuitively to whatever the musical situation calls for—to be sensitive and subtle, then musically bombastic and aggressive. The interplay between great musicians exists solely in the realm of intuition. Just listen to Don Cherry and Ornette Coleman's recording of "Lonely Woman" and the way the two play the melody together, intuitively responding to one another.

The musical equivalent of the intuitive double-play duo of Omar Vizquel and Roberto Alomar was singer Billie Holiday and tenor saxophonist Lester Young. They had worked together for years—Lester Young called Billie Holiday "Lady Day," and she in turn called him "Prez"—and the music they made together was achingly beautiful and perfectly in sync. It was breathtaking.

In one of the great moments in jazz history, the two performed together on a December 5, 1957, CBS television special called "The Sound of Jazz," in which Holiday sang her own song "Fine and Mellow." When "Prez" joined in, a reviewer wrote, "They seemed to anticipate the other's movements just before they happened. Their musical lines flitted and flapped around one another, and occasionally they flew side by side." It remains one of the great live, recorded moments in jazz.

## BEHIND THE INTUITIVE ARTIST (PART TWO)

by Don Greene

Take a more in-depth look at the left and right hemispheres and whole brain functioning. The left brain thinks with words and numbers, and is used in logic and mathematics, in technical and analytical terms. The left brain separates and divides, judges and criticizes, blames and argues, in noisy, high-speed thinking. It thinks in linear terms in the limited dimension of two: plus or minus, black or white, up or down, here or there, past and future, and your choice is to take it or leave it.

The right brain thinks with images, sounds, and sensations, often much quieter and at a slower pace. The right brain thinks in three dimensions: beyond black and white to shades of gray, not to mention the colors of the visible spectrum; as well as here, there, and the space between; in the timeless and unlimited dimension of now beyond words; and your options are to accept it, leave it, or change it.

The left brain is helpful in the early phases of learning athletic, musical, or technical skills. It is an essential part of practice and preparation for actual performances. However, in performance situations, it often gets in the way. The left brain's doubts, worries, criticism, analysis, and judgments cause suboptimal performance. After a suboptimal performance, the left hemisphere blames outside sources for the result it caused, sustaining the unconscious problem.

The right brain is best for imagining possibilities, feeling flowing movements, and hearing the music the way you'd like it to sound. The right hemisphere harmonizes, synthesizes, and integrates distinct parts into wholes without words. The right brain is the source of our intuitive and creative abilities, and a key ingredient in achieving optimal and peak-performance states.

However, both sides of the brain are necessary to produce desired results in reality. The whole brain is required, but it's best used in the correct sequence for specific skills. Athletic and musical skills need to be learned early on through left-brain explanations before they can be executed correctly and felt. But after they're mastered, they are best performed in right-brain quiet without unnecessary instructions or comments.

Leading up to a performance or athletic event, the functional sequence is from left brain to right. The clear intention of the desired result needs to be stated in specific terms and then quietly imagined. A few instructive reminders and positive self-talk can be helpful beforehand, but they become distractions from the right brain's vision, hearing, feeling, and awareness after beginning.

# 6
# Deceptive Cadences

## How positive deception is used in baseball and music

*A deception that elevates us is dearer
than a host of low truths.*

—MARINA TSVETAEVA, RUSSIAN POET

In music, there are chord progressions known as "deceptive cadences"–you think the tune is about to end, and suddenly, the chord change is unexpected and you're in new territory. Music has a lot of positive deception built into it.

The Beatles were masters of positive deception. Whereas nearly every rock, classical, jazz, or country tune written exists in four- or eight-bar phrases, the Beatles turned that notion on its head. Take the song "Yesterday," which every Beatles fan knows. The first phrase of the song is:

> *Yesterday*
> *All my troubles seemed so far away*
> *Now it looks as though they're here to stay*
> *Oh, I believe*
> *In yesterday*

What's deceptive about this, when you listen to it, is that the phrase sounds so natural and right. Yet it isn't the standard four or eight bars. The Beatles created an unheard of phrase in the annals of pop music–a seven-bar phrase. It sounds deceptively simple, but trust us, it's difficult to write a melody that fits within seven bars and make it sound natural. But the Beatles did so masterfully.

If you sing the lyrics a few times, you'll notice that the

phrase is broken down further into sub-phrases. "Yesterday" is a one-bar phrase, after which "All my troubles seemed so far away" is its own two-bar phase, followed by a four-bar phrase: "Now it looks as though they're here to stay, oh, I believe in yesterday." This last four-bar phrase would be normal, especially if it were preceded by another four-bar phrase. But because Paul McCartney is a genius songwriter, that last phrase feels a bit because it's beginning after three bars of music, not four. The melody is perfect–a masterwork of deceptive symmetry built into an odd seven-bar phrase of music.

And that's the hook in the song–a seven-bar phrase broken into asymmetrical sub-phrases that sounds natural when it is anything but. Mozart didn't even do that. The marriage of words, music, and the starts and stops of the phrases is pure genius.

Deception has a negative connotation to it–but not in music. And it shouldn't in baseball either. The game is based on deception, some of it comical. George Bell, who played for the Toronto Blue Jays, would come to the plate and would purposely look foolish on early pitches, leading everyone to think he was not in sync. Then the pitcher would throw a fastball and–boom! Or what about Mickey Rivers, who would drag his feet as he walked into the batter's box, looking out of sorts. Maybe a batter will call time out, acting like something's in their eye, deceiving the pitcher into thinking, "Okay, I can get this guy!" On the contrary, if you're going to bat with a 102-degree fever, or you're injured, you want to act as if you're feeling great.

Derek Jeter endured some calls for an Oscar nomination in the summer of 2010, when a pitch careened off the end of his bat, and Jeter shook his arm enough from the sting that the home-plate umpire thought he was hit by the pitch. But how many times has a player held up his glove with confidence, trying to win an out call on a tag he missed, or the batter who backs away out of the strike zone on a pitch that's over the inside corner, trying to convince the ump it was about to hit him? It's as much a part of the game as a costumed rock guitarist in six-inch heels, jumping off a riser onto the stage as he strikes the proverbial "E-power chord" with his hand, sending the audience into a frenzy. Without the amplification, the costume, the shoes, and–the deception–it would be comical.

The game of baseball is based primarily on the art of positive deception. It tries to make you believe something is real when it's not. A lot of music is based on positive deception too–in fact, if music and baseball didn't deceive, they'd be boring. The Beatles tune "Yesterday" would lose its hook, and baseball would lose its sinker.

The beauty of baseball and music lies in the ability to deceive you about what's really happening. Deception in baseball is a prerequisite, and is paradoxically one of the purest aspects of the game. Outwitting the batter by fooling them with a change-up is a time-honored tradition for pitchers. Without deception, concealment, camouflage, and the antics that go along with it, baseball would become mundane. Imagine if pitchers were required to announce their pitches to the ump before every pitch–how boring (and strange) would that be?!

There is no place where deception is relished more than on the pitcher's mound. A great pitcher can fool the best of hitters, and that's their job–to deceive the batter and so disrupt his timing that he's swinging at what he thinks will be a ninety-five-miles-an-hour fastball when it's simply an eighty-mile-an-hour changeup. But pitchers need to vary the speed only a little bit to create a startling difference between where the batter expects the ball to be and where it actually appears.

In a 2008 article by Adam Summers in *Natural History* magazine, Summers explored the work of two researchers (Terry Bahill, a systems engineer at the University of Arizona, and David Baldwin, a former major-league relief pitcher with an engineering degree and a Ph.D. in genetics) that examined the effect of minute deceptions and change in speed a fastball would have on a hitter.

For example, a few ninety mph fastballs set up the batter to expect more of the same heaters. If the next pitch is 5.5 percent faster, at ninety-five miles per hour, the ball will appear at its point of impact with the bat three inches above where the slower pitch would have. A batter, using a mental model to follow the ball, perceives that as a sudden leap upward as the ball comes back into his region of focus.

That perceptual jump can also explain the phenomenon of the diving curve. While a curve ball certainly does curve, some curve balls appear to the batter to behave quite badly. Players often say, "That one rolled off a table," to describe a ball that drops, or "breaks hard," just before the plate. Bahill and Baldwin reported that, in this case, the pitcher has fooled the batter into thinking the ball is moving faster than it is, leading to a perceptual drop when the ball appears below where the batter expects it.

There is no greater triumph for a pitcher than watching a batter flail away at a ball that's below or in front of where he thought it would be. It's frustrating for the batter, to be sure, but somewhere in the pitcher's mind, he's snickering with delight at having gotten away with it.

Some pitchers have the ability to hide their cards with the way they pitch. Pedro Martinez threw from a low three-quarter position that hid the ball very well, making it difficult to read his pitches and pick up on his delivery. Mariano Rivera is another great deceiver. His cutter is never where you *think* it will be—batters can only guess at where it might be. It becomes a shell game, and if the pitcher is in control, you'll never end up finding that nut underneath.

Batters have a role in trying to outdo the deception of a pitcher. Different pitchers have different rhythms, and the objective is to disrupt the rhythm of the pitcher to the point where he becomes flustered and either loses the ability to deceive you or makes a mistake. Like a cat and mouse game—with the batter stepping out of the box, and the pitcher stepping off the mound—each is trying to deceive and disrupt one another. It's a beautiful thing to watch.

Pitchers who are not power pitchers rely more on deception, as opposed to power pitchers who have a strict sense of rhythm from which they don't deviate. Power pitchers pitch in 4-bar phrases, whereas a deceptive pitcher's rhythm reads more like a 3 or 5-bar phrase. It can throw you off if you're not careful.

The majority of music is "power pitching"–divided neatly into four- or eight-bar phrases. But listen to complex cross-rhythmic music from Eastern Europe–Bulgaria, for example–and you'll encounter asymmetrical rhythms–five-, seven-, nine-, and eleven-bar phrases, along with rhythms that are stilted and awkward, where you are clueless as to when to tap your foot. The great Frank Zappa was a master of this, and his band could play these asymmetrical rhythms with ease. The more asymmetrical you can be in your thinking–and listening to music that is asymmetrical certainly helps–the more you'll be able to react to a deceptive pitcher.

A good example of asymmetrical rhythms in pitching can be found among many of the current pitchers coming out of Japan, like Hideo Nomo, who pitched for the Los Angeles Dodgers. If ever there was a pitcher with an asymmetrical musical windup, it was Nomo. He'd turn his back on the hitter, raise his pivot leg, and freeze for a second before throwing. It was like watching a conductor, his baton in the air, with everyone waiting for the downbeat, but no one has any idea when it's going to come. This asymmetry in his windup was the source of his nickname, "Tornado," and in the 1995 season he led the major leagues in strikeouts, striking out a record 11.1 batters per nine innings to break Sandy Koufax's single-season franchise record, which had stood since 1962.

Pitchers like Nomo have learned to incorporate these deceptively slight hesitations and glitches in their windups that make it difficult for batters to time their swing. They're expecting a four-bar phrase, and then, out of nowhere, comes a 3½-bar phrase. Thus the windup and delivery of a pitcher becomes its own musical phrase–even the rocking back and forth of a pitcher as he gets set has its own musical rhythm to it. The overriding concept, however, is that, as a player, you need to learn the art of positive deception if you're going to rise to the next level.

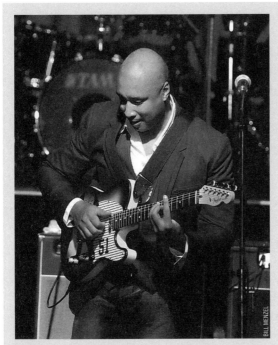

## CHANGE-UP

by Bernie Williams

Jamie Moyer, pitcher for the Seattle Mariners and later the Philadelphia Phillies, was the epitome of deception in a pitcher. He had one of the best changeups in baseball, and he could deceive you with it like no other. I'd be at bat and think, "Okay, here comes his changeup." And I'd be right and then think, "Okay, I know his changeup–now bring it on!" Then he'd throw it again, and I'd think, "Okay, here it is–I see it coming." And I'd be so far out in front of the pitch, because he'd change speeds.

As a guitarist, there's a foot pedal I use called a Limiter–it keeps the sound uniform–not too loud or too soft–and you kinda' expect pitchers to have their own Limiters as well. A changeup is a changeup, right? But not Jaime Moyer! He had no Limiter!

# 7
# Nine-Inning Composition

## How great jazz musicians and ballplayers envision a performance

The great jazz saxophonist John Coltrane had the ability to see across time. Coltrane was a master of jazz improvisation like no other–whereas most jazz musicians improvise thinking conceptually over a four- or eight-bar phrase, Coltrane could, as he began to play, envision his improvisation over the course of an entire solo.

It is rumored that Coltrane would achieve this by practicing playing the chord changes to a song in tempo, on piano, while simultaneously saying the chord changes out loud. He'd go through an entire song like this. But then he'd do something different–he'd repeat playing the chord changes in tempo, but while playing the chord change to the first bar, he'd say the chord change aloud to the second bar. While playing the chord change to the second bar, he'd say the name of the chord in the third bar, and so on.

When he finished this tedious exercise, he'd go back again and play the chord change to the first bar, but say the name of the chord to the third bar, and so on. He would repeat this exercise throughout the entire duration of the tune, such that, if it were a thirty-two-bar song, he'd be playing the chord change to the first bar while saying aloud the chord change to the thirty-second bar! The mental acuity to think ahead and in the moment–to visualize an entire song, a solo, or a game, in that first measure or inning–is a rare talent. But Coltrane evidently possessed it and it certainly showed in his music.

John Coltrane is revered by jazz musicians for bringing jazz to a new plateau—his improvisations transcended the four- and eight-bar-phrase improvisations of the bebop musicians that came before him, taking on an almost spontaneous art of composition. Another artist that has this unique ability to conceptualize over long stretches of time is the gifted jazz pianist Keith Jarrett.

It was January 24, 1975, and Keith Jarrett had not slept in two nights. He was about to make a live recording at the Cologne (Köln) Opera House in Germany, consisting of nothing but solo improvisations. The piano he was supposed to play on—a Bösendorfer 290 Imperial concert grand—was accidently left locked and stored in the cellar of the building. Thus Jarrett had to perform on a tinny and thin-sounding baby grand that was left backstage and in poor condition. The sound engineer decided to go ahead and record the concert, if only for archival purposes. Making matters worse, Jarrett arrived at the opera house late and tired after a long drive in his car. All indications were that the concert would be a disaster. But that's not what happened.

Once Jarrett walked out onstage, everything changed. He focused on his craft, creating some of the most inspired improvisations (one part is a stunning twenty-six minutes long). The concert was an amazing success—and the archival recording was subsequently released, going on to become the bestselling solo album in jazz history. The album is called *The Köln Concert.*

The most notable aspect of this concert was Jarrett's ability to create extended improvisations that became spontaneous compositions. Indeed composers, musicologists, and music theorists have studied this concert, scratching their heads as to how Jarrett could conceive improvisations over such an extended period of time.

There is a parallel between Keith Jarrett and John Coltrane—amazing artists able to conceptualize an entire solo or concert—and baseball figures. Great pitchers are the John Coltranes of the sport, able to conceptualize beyond an inning to an entire nine-inning game. A great pitcher, in his first pitch, can conceptualize and set up a framework and expectations for the later innings. He establishes certain parts of the plate–he pitches differently to the same batter each time he's up, keeping him off guard and guessing. A great pitcher will never approach a good hitter the same way twice–just like a great improviser will always play differently each time.

This ability to master the pitching mound or the musical moment is the domain of great pitchers and musicians. Pedro Martinez, when he was pitching for the Boston Red Sox, was a master improviser performing at the level of a John Coltrane. Flip Bondy, of the *New York Daily News*, said of Pedro, "We see only the high art form–we watch the brain and arm in harmonic convergence, disguising 85-mph fastballs as something far more fanciful than their velocity and arc."

Pedro had the game all thought out, and never pitched the same way twice. His style was atypical, relying on many "out" pitches. He threw fastballs of varying speed, cutters, curveballs, and circle changeups, which when combined with his intellect, proved to be overpowering. In his prime, Martinez's fastball was consistently clocked in the ninety-five to ninety-seven mph range–and combined with his devious changeup, mixed with his curveball–he was as dominant a pitcher as the game has seen. The true artistry of Pedro Martinez, however, was in his ability to use all these pitches to envision a composition that was nine movements–or innings–that began with his very first pitch. Seattle Mariner John Mabry said it best: "If the Lord could pitch, I think he'd be a lot like Pedro."

# JUST ONE SWING

........................................................................................................

by Bernie Williams

........................................................................................................

I can relate to Keith Jarrett not having slept for two nights before a big concert. Professional musicians and ballplayers have to perform at a high level despite illness or a lack of sleep—and deliver. In my sixteen-year career, perhaps 25 percent of the time I wasn't feeling 100 percent—yet I had to give 100 percent of what I did have. Motivation can override all the negatives. In fact, the negatives can become a positive, motivational force.

How you feel before walking onstage or onto the field can have little bearing on the performance. In fact, the opposite can happen: the lack of optimal conditions can be a catalyst for greatness. Baseball players are a superstitious bunch—sometimes in a big game, you'd hope that you'd be feeling lousy and having some minor nagging pain—because it would motivate you to overcome it and do something extraordinary.

Everything that happens to you in your career—both the positive and the negative—can make you a better musician or ballplayer if you channel it correctly. If I was in a slump while playing the Red Sox at Fenway, and the crowd was screaming for me to strike out, I'd use the slump and the crowd as a positive channel to fuel my motivation and desire to get a hit.

One of the best moments where a player channeled the negative into a positive was Game 1 of the 1988 World Series, between the Dodgers and Athletics. With a bad left hamstring and a swollen right knee, Kirk Gibson hobbled up to the plate to pinch-hit in the bottom of the ninth, two men out, with the Dodgers trailing, 4–3, and a runner on first. In one of the most stirring wins in baseball history, Gibson hit a home run, winning the game for the Dodgers. It would be his only plate appearance in the series, and that home run from an injured Gibson motivated the Dodgers, who were the underdogs, to go on and win their sixth World Series.

Fortune can change with just one swing.

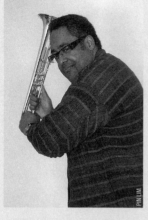

## SWINGING FOR THE FENCES

by Jon Faddis, trumpeter extraordinaire, who performed with Dizzy Gillespie, Paul Simon, and on hundreds of records and sound tracks, as well as directing the Carnegie Hall Jazz Band

There have been three things I learned from great baseball players: be relaxed, be focused, and always sit next to someone more experienced than you.

The Count Basie Band's concept of music is a great example for musicians and ballplayers. It was powerful but relaxed—it didn't matter how fast or slow the music was, it was always relaxed. As a musician, as soon as you tense up, the ideas stop flowing and you cease to be creative, just as you would be in the batter's box. That's why when you'd watch Joe Morgan and he's swinging the bat back and forth, he's doing it to stay relaxed.

Ted Williams is a great example of a ballplayer who had intense focus—it was uncanny. I learned a lot as a musician from watching him play baseball, and tried to be as focused on the bandstand as he was at the plate.

The one thing that is common among ballplayers and musicians is the concept of mentorship. Older players will take younger players under their wings and help them along. This was especially helpful to me when I was on the road as a young kid—you'd get on the bus, and there was someone to mentor you. I was incredibly fortunate to have a mentor like no other—the great Dizzy Gillespie. Dizzy would take me aside and say, "Look, this is how it's done." It was an incredible experience and one of the reasons that I teach—to return to others what Dizzy gave to me. Seeking out a mentor, whether it's a Don Zimmer or a Dizzy Gillespie, is crucial for young players.

One of the things that Dizzy Gillespie said about bebop was that bebop musicians make each other sound better. That's the goal of bebop and that's what great ballplayers do too—try to make everyone else play and look good.

The beauty of baseball and jazz today is that it doesn't matter who you are, where you're from, the color of your skin—jazz and baseball embrace everyone, and you're respected solely on the basis of what you can do on the field or on the bandstand.

# 8
# Anticipation

How to develop rhythmic acuity

*We won't get fooled again.*
−THE WHO

*Anticipation, anticipation*
*Is makin' me late*
*Is keepin' me waitin'*
−CARLY SIMON

It is one of the most awkward, embarrassing moments on the field or on the stage. Whether you're a ballplayer or a musician, you've had it happen to you. Go on, admit it–you were at bat and you sensed a fastball coming and swung ridiculously early on a changeup. You got fooled–again. Or maybe you misread the downbeat from the conductor and came in early and everyone–*everyone*–notices. Whether it happens on the field or on the stage, the world stops, your body wilts, your mind is in disarray, and your focus is shot.

Experienced musicians rarely get fooled again–they've developed their timing to such a degree that these embarrassing episodes rarely occur. Experienced ballplayers rarely get fooled either, especially by inexperienced pitchers–but put an ace on the mound who can wreak havoc with a player's timing–and all bets are off.

To put it in perspective, consider this: the distance from the pitcher's mound to the plate is sixty feet six inches. A ninety-five-mile-an-hour fastball travels at 139.33 feet every second. It takes only .434 seconds from the time the ball leaves the pitcher's glove until it reaches the plate. Yet, the batter has to react in half that time–roughly .2 seconds in order to prepare to swing. Hitting a ninety-five-mile-an-hour fastball is perhaps one of the hardest things to do (and even if you're very successful at it by major league standards, you'll still fail every seven out of ten times!). But the batter's box isn't the only place where this level of reaction time is required: musicians responding to the split-second downbeat of a conductor require this same reaction time as well.

Great musicians and great ballplayers have an intuitive rhythmic sense of what's going to happen in that next fraction of a second. Younger musicians and ballplayers need to learn to intuit what's going to happen in that fraction of a second before it does. This rhythmic acuity is often called "playing in the zone". It can't be taught, but it can be learned. Let's try this experiment:

Sit with a friend with your backs opposite one another so that you cannot see each other's hands or face. Count off aloud, "One-two-three-four," in rhythm (each beat should be about a second) and begin clapping together. Keep clapping until you both feel like you're rhythmically locked in and in sync with one another. Now, here's the hard part: While still clapping in rhythm, count aloud, "One-two-three-four," and stop clapping on beat "five," but silently continue counting (five-six-seven-eight-nine-ten-eleven-twelve-thirteen-fourteen) in rhythm. When you reach beat "fifteen," both of you clap aloud. What happened? Were you in sync? Did one of you come in too late or early? Repeat the exercise and try to focus on locking in both of your internal rhythms. If it still proves too difficult, try a lower number (for example, count only to eight or ten).

What you may notice in doing this exercise is that your mind starts to behave differently. You're focused, locked in, and concentrating on that internal rhythm that you both generated aloud through clapping. With no audible information, you have to rely entirely on your intuition and internal rhythm. When you're totally focused and internalizing the rhythm, and you both clap at the same point after a period of silence, you're both locked into the zone.

Great musicians and great ballplayers have this ability

to lock into the zone. A good example of this is in jazz—especially free jazz, where there may not be any predetermined tempo, requiring the musicians to lock into each other's rhythms and style. Great free jazz musicians—like Ornette Coleman, Pat Metheny, and John Coltrane—are not unlike a batter focused and locked into the zone, responding intuitively off of a pitcher. The great free jazz musicians of baseball are players like Derek Jeter, Vladimir Guerrero, and Ichiro Suzuki, who have the ability to lock into the zone and respond to whatever situation they are in.

Why is this ability important? When you're at the plate, you need to try to internalize the rhythms of the pitcher and anticipate what's going to happen in that two-tenths of a second before you start your swing. Many young batters start their swings too early trying to anticipate the pitch, and they lose the zone and are out ahead of the pitch. Once you've started your swing, there's no turning back: you've lost all hope of applying power to your swing. However, if you keep your hands back for as long as you can and focus, you'll have a much better chance at making contact.

The key here is timing. It's unlikely that, when the pitch actually comes, your timing will be perfectly in sync, as it's unlikely you'll know exactly what that pitch will be. But by keeping your hands back and allowing yourself time to react, you'll have force to apply to the swing even if you've mistimed the pitch and your rhythm isn't in sync with the pitcher. But if your hands come forward too quickly, you'll get fooled on the pitch and have no power in your swing.

The important point here is that, by waiting and keeping your hands back, you can compensate for the lack of time, because you don't have to hit the ball straight, you can pull it or hit it the other way.

In this way, the batter's box or strike zone, for an instant, is analogous to a rhythmic beat. You can play ahead of the beat (swing early) or you can play behind the beat (swing too late). But there's room to maneuver in that beat (the batter's box).

The Count Basie Band swung like no other band in history, and the way they played was to play on the back part of the beat (analogous to keeping your hands back and swinging at the last possible moment). A symphony orchestra, however, is likely to play at the front part of the beat (analogous to swinging the bat either at exactly the precise moment needed to drive the ball straight or a bit early). It's best, though, to think like a jazz musician–like Count Basie–and keep your hands back. You'll be in a better position to react and make contact.

For musicians, a great way to develop this rhythmic skill is to practice improvising with another person (don't worry–you don't have to be a jazz musician to do this–just make up whatever comes into your head). As you and your fellow musician are improvising, be sure you're focused on what the other person is playing and see how you can relate what you're playing to what the other person is doing. At first, the exercise might seem awkward–even silly–but keep focusing. What will emerge after much practice is a higher level of awareness and intuition–you're likely to discover that, even though you don't know what the other person is about to play, you'll be intuitively anticipating and responding to it, much like a great hitter would. You'll also be amazed at how your awareness and focus is heightened. Great jazz musicians have this heightened focus and awareness–and so do great hitters. The mindset is virtually the same.

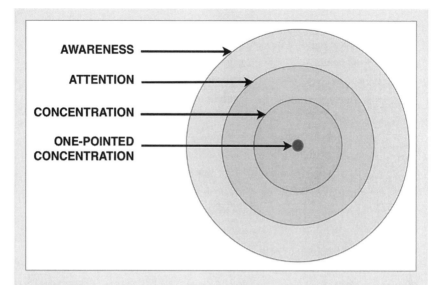

# FOCUS

by Don Greene

Concentration is a right-brain, alpha state of mental quiet. It is free from distracting left-brain words and analysis. There are several different mindsets in performing jazz and playing baseball; they are best understood as a series of concentric circles.

The outer circle is awareness. It is the knowledge of what is happening in the immediate environment around you and also inside you. Awareness is the outer ring.

When you focus your awareness, you begin to pay attention. Attention is the next ring. You focus on one thing at a time as you smoothly shift to the correct type of attention for the demands of the ever-changing situation.

When you focus your full attention in the here and now, you move past external and internal distractions to the third ring. The innermost ring is concentration. You become totally absorbed in the moment with the task at hand to the exclusion of all else.

When you become one with the object of your focus, you achieve one-pointed concentration. This is the central point of the concentric circles: it is the bull's-eye. It involves a merging of subject, tool, and object: archer, bow, and target; musician, instrument, and music; and batter, bat, and ball.

Concentration requires an enormous amount of energy. Make sure that you get sufficient rest before live performances or games, so you can accumulate the energy necessary to stay focused. It takes energy just to pay attention. You're less alert when you're tired, and able to focus much better when you're fresh and rested.

Although it takes a lot of energy to focus properly, concentration is not a forced state. It is a state of effortless power, allowing that powerful energy to flow effortlessly into the object of your focused attention. The process is not a doing as much as an allowing yourself to be fully with something. This total mindfulness is like lovers beholding their beloved.

Have a routine that you follow before you play that prepares you to focus exclusively on the task at hand for the required period of time. When you find your attention straying, which it will, simply bring it back to the task at hand without delay or frustration.

Learn how to quiet your left-brain noise and shift to the quiet right brain before you begin playing or performing. You can do this by hearing the sound you'd like to create, seeing the image of making a good play, or the feeling of hitting a homerun.

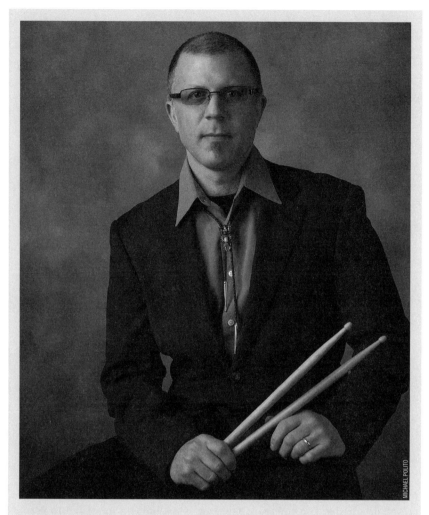

MICHAEL POLITO

# PRACTICING WITH DISTRACTIONS

by Dave Gluck

It might seem counterintuitive, but it's actually very helpful for musicians to develop their concentration and focus by including distractions in their practicing, not unlike a major leaguer on the road who has to block out the less than encouraging home crowd when he's at bat. Think about it: ballplayers have to perform under the loudest of distractions—50,000 fans screaming for you to strike out. Musicians practice and perform in the sanctuary of a practice room or a concert hall, where the audience, unlike at a ball game, is not even supposed to cough.

From early on, young ballplayers get used to performing regularly with distractions, yet young musicians seldom get to perform in public as often as their Little League counterparts. For the first timer, the mere sight of a packed recital hall can distract, simply because, after so many months of practice, there are now people in the room—which, even though they're quiet, can be unnerving and distracting if you haven't properly prepared for it.

In my senior year as a music major at Ithaca College, my professor suggested that I purposely practice with distractions so that I could learn to focus and concentrate on making better music. My junior recital had gone well, but I found myself out of focus and distracted, unable to fully concentrate on the music. He suggested I bring a boom box into the practice room, set the dial to a news or sports show, turn up the volume, and play. It was a strange, counterintuitive experience—at first, it was impossible to concentrate on the music without getting lost in the box scores from the previous night's games. But after a week, I began to tolerate it and even make music alongside it. My sense of 'tunnel-hearing' became more acute, and I began to block out the radio. As my level of focus improved, I found I could allow my mind to absorb the sounds of the radio when I wanted, without it distracting from my practice. In essence, I developed the ability to "double-task" and it significantly improved my performance level in concerts.

This is a skill that musicians seldom practice—yet great ballplayers have all acquired it. The difference, however, is that unlike a hitter at the plate blocking out a roaring crowd, a musician needs to paradoxically focus on "hitting the ball" while simultaneously engaging the audience. This bifurcated ability to be simultaneously in the music and with the audience is the hallmark of great musicians.

# 9
# Mental Preparedness

## How to prepare for performance

*I have yet to be in a game where luck was involved. Well-prepared players make plays. I have yet to be in a game where the most prepared team didn't win.*
–URBAN MEYER, FOOTBALL COACH

*Despair is most often the offspring of ill-preparedness.*
–DON WILLIAMS JR., AMERICAN NOVELIST AND POET

Early on in my career with the Yankees, when I first came up to the major leagues, I tried to control what I could not. In baseball, perhaps more than any other sport, players make feeble attempts to control what they absolutely have no control over. The game is filled with variables that change, evolve, and devolve every inning and every second. Yet the rhythms of the game remain the same: players move in and out in the exactly the same way as they have done for over a century. This is baseball's paradox: there is chaos within order, and order within chaos.

There exists no other team sport where the dimensions of the playing field change from stadium to stadium and can have a huge impact on the game (think "Green Monster" at Fenway Park). Pitchers, batters, and umpires change–fans even sound different from game to game. No two umpires set the strike zone exactly the same, and thus no two games are alike. The only visual constant on the field is the shape of the diamond and nine players on the field. Despite the symmetry and order of baseball's rules, the game never feels the same–

and when things never feel the same, there is the potential to be distracted–to let the variables influence you to a point where you're in chaos. This is the essence of baseball when it's played at its highest level.

No one who takes the field should assume anything, and nothing should be taken for granted. Experienced players know that anything can happen at any time. Time is not a factor in baseball–you can't wear down your opponent and win a game with the clock. In this way, baseball is very elusive and very unpredictable, like Ornette Coleman playing free jazz.

The players that try to control baseball's chaos fail dramatically. You can see the frustration in their eyes and by how they react. They've tried to control the chaos around them, and chaos won. It's impossible to control chaos and change, so don't even attempt it–those that do only lead themselves down a rabbit hole that is counterproductive and, for some, self-destructive. More importantly, when a player gets frustrated, he's not focusing and concentrating, which leads to distraction. And when you're distracted, you're not going to be at your best.

Baseball was designed to be distracting, frustrating, and elusive. No other sport invokes you to fail more often than succeed. A musician missing seven out of every ten notes would get booed off the stage (or off of *Guitar Hero!*), but in baseball, batting .300 means you're doing very well, by failing 70 percent of the time! This is baseball's gift to us–that only through failing can we ultimately succeed. It is one of the reasons why music has influenced how I played baseball. The greatest performing musicians of all time–from jazz saxophonist John Coltrane to guitarist Eric Clapton to the classical cellist Yo-Yo Ma–have this uncanny ability and talent to achieve perfection and excellence at a level far beyond the dreams of any ballplayer.

Think about it: Yo-Yo Ma's batting average, playing the Dvorak Cello Concerto with the New York Philharmonic is at least .980! Thousands of variables lay before him as he walks out onstage–the notes, the rhythms, the tempi, the orchestra, the conductor, etc. Yet somehow he is able to focus and channel all this into a performance that is closer to perfection than any batter could ever hope.

Confronted with the odds stacked against you when you go to the plate–playing a game "that is more varied than any dance"–how do you bring order to it all? The answer is twofold: thorough preparation and a solid mental approach to the game. These are the only two things you can ultimately control, and it is something that every great artist has in their arsenal when they walk onstage or onto the field.

The mark of a great ballplayer is one who takes the field thoroughly prepared and defined in their approach with the goal of "succeeding utterly." Part of that approach is playing the game hard–with a level of concentration that would rival that of a skilled concert violinist. Great players understand this–there is no clock in baseball, and you play hard until the very last out is made.

If you prepare thoroughly, and approach the game consistently, you will weather every low and temper every high. The results will be the effect, not the cause, of your success, for your success will have its foundation built upon a rock of preparedness and approach.

I can't overemphasize this enough to young ballplayers and musicians. There is no short cut, as I learned from studying guitar in my youth: you have to prepare thoroughly–no matter how naturally talented you may be–and you have to translate that preparedness into a solid mental approach. The players with the most successful, enduring careers–like Cal Ripken, Jr.–have this level of preparedness and approach. For me, the work ethic of players like this is what is truly inspiring and great about the game.

The great players who have done extraordinary things in clutch situations may not have all shared the same natural talent and ability early on. But there is one thing they did share–they were prepared for those extraordinary moments when the chance was given to them to do extraordinary things. It's no accident–and certainly, luck plays a part. But at the foundation of every amazing and historic play lies solid preparation coupled with a sound mental approach that made the moment possible.

Preparation is the fuel that drives great artists and musicians. The countless hours spent practicing alone–whether in a practice room or on the field–are like deposits in a bank that accumulate over time to be drawn upon in those moments when we are summoned to do the heroic. Preparation gives you confidence and a sense of self-worth in your craft. It gives you peace of mind during dark days, and the fortitude to accept whatever the results or consequences may be.

Losing takes on a different tone and perspective when you know you were fully prepared–you will learn from it and improve. And of course, there is no greater feeling than having prepared thoroughly for the moment and responding to it in a way that brought out the best of you and your years of training. But there is no worse feeling than being unprepared for the moment and failing in anger or despair.

Great ballplayers also understand that physical preparation can only work if one has developed a solid, consistent mental approach to playing the game. Think about it: baseball is unique in that the amount of time a ball is in play represents very little time within the game itself. Most of the time on the field is spent anticipating, preparing, strategizing, focusing, and then–and only then–executing a play in a matter of seconds. Before every play, players are concentrating, trying to anticipate, ensuring they are prepared for every variable.

The most successful ballplayer has conceived of a sound mental approach to the game. It is the least talked about part of playing baseball. Young players often devote their focus to the mechanics–hitting, fielding, and executing plays–but it is in reality one's mental approach, combined with thorough physical preparedness, that will ultimately determine whether they are successful.

My approach before every game was to begin that game in complete neutrality and consistency in my attitude and approach. This entailed not letting the highs (hitting a walk-off home run in the last game) or the lows (striking out the night before) enter too far into my psyche that it either altered my mental concentration or neutrality to begin the game anew. The only way I could achieve this was through the ritual of practice and approach.

When I first signed with the Yankees, my agent, Scott Boras, imparted some invaluable words to me: "Prepare well and let the results be what they may." In a sport that is so focused on results and statistics, the advice might seem out of sync and counterintuitive. It's not: there are only two things you can control in baseball and it is your preparation and your approach.

Beyond solid preparation, how does one develop the right mental approach to the game? How does one mentally prepare for the next series, game, inning, and play? The secret lies in reducing variables.

Baseball is a complex game with a seemingly infinite set of variables. But in any one given situation, you can limit, refine, and distill those variables down to a manageable number. On the field, the time spent with the ball not in play is when you have the opportunity to hone your approach, reduce the variables in the given situation, and execute your plan of attack. There are hundreds of variables involved before every play, but the more you've done your homework and refined your approach, the less insurmountable those variables will seem.

There are variables—but they are not infinite.

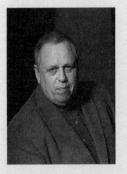

## EFFORTLESS MASTERY

by Kenny Werner, jazz pianist and composer, author of the book, *Effortless Mastery—Liberating the Master Musician Within*

*It is good to view things as familiar or unfamiliar, rather than as difficult or easy. If you give yourself the message, "this is difficult," the piece may discourage you and it will still be difficult to play even after you've learned it. However, if you believe that all music is easy, then you'll assume that you are unfamiliar with the piece because "it hasn't become easy yet."*

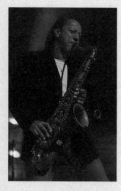

## READINESS

by Richie Cannata, saxophonist with Bernie Williams, Billy Joel, the Beach Boys, and many others

*You can't come off the bench and not be ready—you can't say, "Coach, I didn't know I was going to pinch-hit, I'm not ready." Likewise, young musicians need to be ready and prepared when they get the call for that big gig. This is the moment that musicians and athletes live for—where pre-paredness and opportunity meet. As a professional musician or ballplayer, you have to prepare so thoroughly that, even on a bad day, you still perform at a very high level.*

# 10
# Reducing Variables

## How reducing variables improves your performance

*You take as many variables out of your game as possible, and it helps turn the percentages more in your favor.*
−MARK LORETTA

*One man's constant is another man's variable.*
−ALAN PERLIS

*The circumstances of the world are so variable that an irrevocable purpose or opinion is almost synonymous with a foolish one.*
−WILLIAM SHAKESPEARE

One of the most important concepts I learned while playing with the Yankees was how to reduce variables. The game of baseball is comprised of controllable and uncontrollable factors. The controllable factors are your preparation and your approach, while the uncontrollable factors are everything else, including the players, the umpires, the weather, the fans, and anything that you can imagine.

Game 2 of the 2007 ALCS in Cleveland between the Indians and the Yankees showed everyone yet another unexpected variable. It seems that every fall, swarms of harmless (they don't bite) mosquito-like insects leave their homes along the shores of Lake Erie looking for action and bright lights. On October 5 of that year, they found it−descending like a swarm onto Progressive Field in Cleveland, wreaking havoc on the Yankees and pitcher Joba Chamberlain. But other than bringing a can of OFF! to the ballpark with you, it's simply not a variable over which anyone has much control.

Reducing variables is a key component of a great player's mental approach to the game. It involves as much work for your mind as physical preparation demands from your body, and yet many young players neglect this vital component in their development. The reduction of variables in any situation depends on the amount of mental "homework" you've done studying your opponent, combined with your ability to intuitively act on what you've learned. Great players have a deep well of knowledge and experience to draw on too, and are thus able to further reduce the variables. The goal, however, is to never walk onto the field or take an at bat in which there exists variables that you could have eliminated through preparation and study. Ever.

To give you a prime example, the simplest way to reduce variables during an at bat is to bunt. Inherently designed to reduce variables, bunting enables the batter to make contact with the ball with the hopes of advancing the runner. A bunt requires a certain action on the hitter's part–to simply allow the ball to make contact with the bat–and that action reduces the variables. Another example is when you're in a sacrifice-fly situation–let's say there is a runner on second with no one out. Your primary responsibility is to move the runner over by hitting the ball to the right side. You usually use the first two strikes to attempt this, reducing the variables. If you're not successful, then you need to expand the variables and do whatever you can to make it a successful at bat.

When a batter faces a pitcher, the batter should be able to reduce the variables through learning about the pitcher's repertoire and pitching style. If you know that the pitcher throws a fastball, slider, and curve, you can reduce the variables by knowing that he won't likely be throwing you a changeup. You've eliminated a variable. Further, if you've done your homework and know the stats on the pitcher and how he throws to batters like you, you can reduce the variables even further, perhaps eliminating certain portions of the strike zone. If it's a crucial game situation, a pitcher will likely never throw anything but his best pitch–the pitch that got him into the majors—and thus in a crucial situation, you can paradoxically reduce the variables even further still.

Knowing how the specific pitch count will influence the pitcher is also crucial in reducing the variables. Obviously, if you have two strikes on you, you have no choice but to expand the strike zone, thus creating more variables. But if the pitch count is in your favor, you can be more selective: you can pick your zone within the three-dimensional strike zone. Then, if the ball is in that zone, a good hitter will simply not miss it. Eliminating sections within the strike zone is a key way to reduce variables.

A batter has the uncertainty of not knowing when the pitcher will make a mistake—however, a batter can eliminate one variable—the pitcher *will* eventually make a mistake. After all, pitchers aren't machines. But the real issue for the batter is, "When will the pitcher make that mistake?" And when that mistake happens, is the batter fully prepared and focused to take advantage of that opportunity?

Of course, there are days when pitchers are "on their game," pitching perfectly, and a batter really has no chance of making decent contact with the ball. This is how the game was designed, and it hasn't changed. Don Larsen's perfect game pitching in the 1956 World Series versus the Brooklyn Dodgers stands out as a remarkable achievement. On that day, reducing the variables was impossible for the hitter—when a pitcher is perfect, the only thing you can do is tip your hat and applaud.

In addition to reducing variables on offence, there are opportunities to reduce variables on defense as well. When I was playing in an unfamiliar ballpark, I would actually go out and throw balls against the center-field wall to see how they would bounce. I'd look at the turf and see how the cut of the grass would affect how fast or slow a ball would roll. If you're playing in left or right field, it's vital that you get used to the corners. Some stadiums have more foul territory than others, and you need to be prepared for that.

The time of day, weather, and which way the stadium is facing can help you reduce variables. When I played in Oakland against the A's at Alameda County Coliseum, the sun and sky could be treacherous, and you'd lose all perspective on a high fly ball–it was like trying to spot a spec of dust a hundred feet high. Knowing that information up front helped me reduce variables.

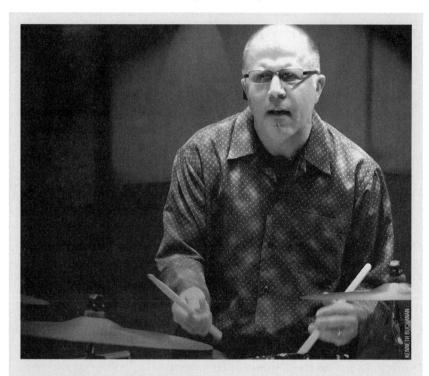

## VARIABLES IN MUSIC

by Dave Gluck

Musicians employ two approaches to reducing variables that mirror those in baseball: isolation and "incrementalization." Isolation involves separating a musical passage (from a single note or gesture to an entire phrase) and focusing repeatedly on perfecting it. This is part of the reason you hear musicians practicing scales constantly–scales form the basis of all melodies, and if you've perfected these scales, then playing any musical passage becomes all that much easier. Scales are akin to calisthenics in baseball. All great musicians practice them, regardless of whether they play mainly classical, jazz, rock, etc.

Incrementalization centers on the tempo and length of the passage that a musician is practicing. Once you have isolated the musical excerpt or technique you wish to focus on, you can begin working at a slow enough tempo so that you can play that passage without mistakes. Musicians often use a metronome to practice incrementalization, starting sometimes at a painfully slow tempo and gradually, through many repetitions, working it up to performance tempo. The important element in incrementalization is to move the tempo up slowly, so that the increment is minute. This allows your muscle memory time to adjust. Here's an example:

Let's say I'm working on a highly intricate groove pattern on the drum set that involves complex contributions from all four limbs (and one brain that acts as central command, hopefully). The pattern with all of its permutations is sixteen measures in length and ultimately needs to be played at 140 beats per minute (bpm). Perhaps I'll start by isolating (and looping) only the first two measures of the pattern, choosing a tempo slow enough (i.e., perhaps half speed at 70 bpm) so that I have complete command of my actions, both mentally and physically. I'll practice the first two measures like this until I'm in what baseball players call "the zone"—where it feels entirely comfortable, effortless, and natural. Then I'll increase the tempo by a miniscule increment—perhaps from 70 bpm to 72 bpm—an increase that doesn't tax my brain and muscles. I'll keep increasing the tempo like this, slowly and laboriously, until I've gotten the tempo up to 140 bpm. The result is that, when I finally can play the passage at 140 bpm, my muscle memory and mind are solidly in control, and I can begin to involve myself more creatively in the musical aspects of the passage.

This works for ballplayers too: practicing hitting a ball that is slowly soft tossed (underhand) allows you to focus on the mechanics of your swing. Gradually, you can work up to the speed of the pitch. There is no way anyone can hit a ninety-five-mile-an-hour fastball without first learning how to hit one that is thrown ninety miles an hour. In the batting cages, most young ballplayers gravitate to the fast-pitch cage. It's far better to start with the slow pitch first, and achieve mastery of it before you move up in speed.

Even if you can already hit a fastball (regardless of the speed), you might reverse the process and start to slow the speed of the pitch down incrementally. If I can play a passage at a fast tempo, I'll sometimes work backwards with it, slowing the passage down more and more with each repetition to the point where I'm playing the passage at half speed. This is a marvelous way to learn and master a musical passage, such that when you're playing it at a fast tempo, you have total control over it, regardless of the tempo. Often times I'll find that by slowing down a passage, I'll uncover some weaknesses or flaws in my technique that weren't evident when I was playing at a fast tempo. Practicing slowly is a musician's equivalent of practicing hitting with the ball on the tee.

# 11
# The On-Off Switch

How to develop mental endurance

*There's a lot of wonderful stillness in baseball that I love. Mini-seconds of stillness, when the pitcher has gotten the sign, when the batter is crouched, the players all lean forward with their hands on their knees. And then very shortly the ball is delivered. But in that tiny period when that pitch and fever in the crowd is tangible, there's a moment of absolute stillness that I treasure.*
–DONALD HALL, POET

Early in my career while playing center field, I would often become exhausted mentally because I did not know how to manage my internal "on-off switch." I would concentrate on the game constantly, during the pitch and also in between pitches. Eventually I realized that my mind–my brain is just another muscle and doesn't have the capacity to be holding this mental weight continuously. One of the critical defensive strategies I learned playing in the outfield for the Yankees was this mental on-off switch.

Imagine it's a scorching 103-degree Saturday afternoon in the Bronx, sweltering heat, the sun burning down on the field, and the game is tied, 1–1, going into the sixth inning. You're in center field, sweating, feeling the onslaught of potential heat exhaustion. Many of the fans with seats in the direct sun simply can't take the heat and have headed for shade elsewhere at Yankee Stadium. Your mind is overrun by thoughts of the heat–you're imagining at this moment, if only there were a swimming pool out behind the wall in center, what it would feel like to dive in after the inning is over.

Maybe it's the opposite–you're playing an October playoff

game in thirty-degree light drizzle at the new Target Field in Minnesota, wishing that they had spent that extra money for the retractable roof like they had in the old Metrodome. Regardless, neither situation is ideal for baseball, yet games, pennants, and even World Series are decided in weather like this.

Baseball doesn't require the level of physical endurance and perseverance of a marathon runner, yet it requires a level of continuous concentration for upwards of four hours at a time. It is a mentally strenuous game—make no mistake about it. During the course of a game, there could be as many as 200 pitches, and each pitch requires the defense to be totally focused, alert, and ready to make split-second plays. You may be out in center field in sweltering heat, but your eyes are glued to the pitcher and batter, watching every movement.

When the pitcher begins his windup, you get set, and your center of gravity is such that you can immediately fly in any direction in an instant. You're in expectation mode—time freezes and your focus is so intense at this point that nothing else matters except that ball passing over the plate. And then the pitch is a ball, and you relax for a few seconds, and repeat the process for every pitch. You do this on average 150 times a game, on and off, 162 times a year. Twenty seconds of intense concentration, which over the course of a twenty-four-week regular season adds up to five to seven hours a week spent doing nothing except concentrating intensely, twenty seconds at a time, on and off. It can take its toll, to be sure.

Imagine too what it feels like to spend the entire day in the outfield having seen no action—and it's now the bottom of the ninth and your pitcher has a no-hitter going when suddenly—*crack!* The ball is flying out into center field and the no-hitter hangs entirely on how quickly you can react. For three hours, you've been standing; now you're sprinting like a gazelle.

Baseball is unique in this way—it's perhaps the only sport where defensive players spend the majority of their time concentrating, anticipating, expecting, and strategizing. Great defensive players have impeccable mental concentration—an ability to block everything out and focus on the one thing that matters most: that ball passing over the plate.

It's easier when conditions are good—the weather is optimal, you're feeling great, and you're energized, and those seven hours a week spent watching that ball pass over the plate from 350 feet away are reasonable. But when you're tired, ill, the weather is wreaking havoc, or mosquitoes are having a picnic in the outfield—well, then it requires a level of perseverance that only a Biblical Job could have. Yet great major league players do rise to the occasion day in and day out—and so do musicians.

If you want to witness intense concentration at this level by musicians, look no further than the orchestra pit of the Metropolitan Opera House in New York City. The Metropolitan Opera Orchestra is the busiest orchestra in the country, performing over 200 times a year—and operas at the Met can take on the time duration of a typical Yankees–Red Sox game, lasting upwards of four hours or more. The musicians in this orchestra are among the best in the world, and if you're a violinist in the Met orchestra, you're fortunate to be playing the majority of the time. But not everyone is.

Take for instance the third trumpet player, who might have to count over 100 measures of rest and then play a critical fanfare right at the entrance of a new scene, after which they'll rest for another 40 measures and then play another critical phrase.

Throughout the opera, the majority of the time is spent waiting, counting, focusing, and getting ready to play. The amount of time actually spent playing their instrument throughout the opera might be as little as 5 percent—maybe only twenty minutes total—yet they have to be tuned in and focused virtually all the time. On and off, it goes like this for sometimes as long as four or five hours.

This is a seldom made comparison between the outfield of a major league baseball team and the "outfield"—in this case, the brass section—of a major league opera orchestra. Both the ballplayer and musician in this scenario need to turn the concentration switch on and off, continuously, for hours at a time. So how do you develop the proper approach to this level of concentration over prolonged periods of time? How do you remain focused and ready for when the ball is hit to you? And it *will* be hit to you, eventually!

Every great major league defensive player has an "on-off" mechanism they've developed. When there's no play, it's vital you relax, take your mind off things–even if it's for a few seconds. When you see an outfielder looking up at the stands or the sky in between pitches, you can bet they're not trying to spot a relative or friend–they're purposefully taking their mind off the game for a few seconds, lest they burn out from the intense level of concentration required.

In some ways, playing defense–whether in the infield or outfield, requires a higher level of focus and concentration than hitting. When you're hitting, you're operating at 100 percent with every at bat–but that's maybe a total of only ten to fifteen minutes a game. But there's much more downtime in center field, and many more distractions that can cause your mind to wander–and in places like Fenway, there are a plethora of willing fans to help your mind wander!

There is, however, a fine line between letting your mind relax between pitches to replenish your concentration and getting too distracted and wandering too far from the game. Thus, you not only need this on-off switch: you need to have complete control of it as well.

If you want to see the creative, sometimes hysterical "off-switch" meanderings of an outfielder, you can often find it at your nearest Little League game (the littler the better). The poor center fielder is standing out there in the fields–swatting away bees, chasing after a butterfly, smelling the fresh cut grass–when *crack!* The ball is headed in his or her direction, invading the pastoral serenity of what was center field.

The fielder looks up, bewildered and shocked, and the ball drops somewhere a few yards away. The majority of balls that drop in the outfield during a Little League game are simply because the fielder hadn't developed an on-off switch. In major league baseball, however, there is absolutely no excuse for not being 100 percent ready for that situation when the ball and bat meet.

Another crucial component in developing your on-off switch is that you need an intermediary stop between "on" and "off." In other words, a "standby" mode. A standby mode is somewhere between on and off, and it's where you can be in a semi-relaxed state while visualizing ahead to the next pitch. During standby mode, you need to be dissecting the game situation, reducing the variables, and envisioning what might happen on that next pitch.

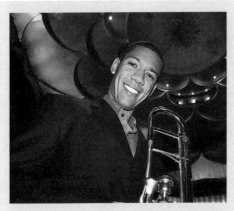

## A NIGHT AT THE OPERA

by Weston Sprott, trombonist with the Metropolitan Opera Orchestra

Members of the trombone section definitely need an on-off switch in order to execute their duties in the orchestra appropriately. I believe a prime example is the opera by composer Richard Wagner, *Die Walküre* (The Valkyries), a five-and-a-half-hour opera that features the famous "Ride of the Valkyries" that has been popularized in everything from the movie *Apocalypse Now* to Elmer Fudd cartoons. The show opens with a driving string bass line that is capped off by the brass who have just counted seventy-two bars of rests. Immediately following this, the trombone section then rests for around half an hour before being called upon to play an extremely delicate, soft chorale. On paper this passage is seemingly simple, but performing it accurately after such a long rest period is significantly more difficult than it appears to the audience. The members of the trombone section recognize this difficulty and breathe a sigh of relief after having done it well and not drawing too much attention to themselves. Just as fans at a baseball game may think nothing of a "routine" out on a pop fly, the outfielder realizes that it only appears to be routine because of hundreds of hours of practice, making sure that he is correctly positioned, acutely focused, and ready to spring into action after minutes, or sometimes hours, of relative inactivity.

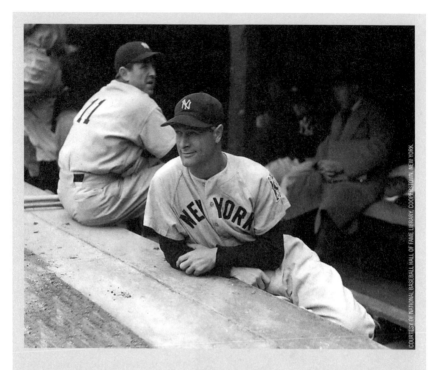

COURTESY OF NATIONAL BASEBALL HALL OF FAME LIBRARY, COOPERSTOWN, NEW YORK.

# A LESSON IN PERSEVERANCE

by Bernie, Dave, and Bob

> *He was a symbol of indestructibility–a Gibraltar in cleats.*
> –Jim Murray, sports columnist, on Lou Gehrig

Developing a solid working on-off switch is key to excelling at defense, and it is also the key to developing your mental and physical perseverance on the field. But there are other factors involved in perseverance as well. If you're ill, if you have a family member who is ill back home and you can't be there to help, or perhaps you're going through a rough time personally–all these important facets of life that you can't neglect are there with you on the field, and you need to find a way to cope.

One of the greatest examples of perseverance among major league ballplayers was Lou Gehrig. Gehrig never thirsted for the limelight. He showed up to work faithfully every day and did his job, and was happy to do so. That some of his teammates–first Babe Ruth, and later Joe DiMaggio–commanded greater attention, didn't bother Gehrig. He said Ruth's big shadow "gave me lots of room to spread myself."

He was nicknamed "Iron Horse," and it's not hard to see why. He played through back pain, broken bones in his toes and fingers—in fact, his doctors later found evidence of seventeen different hand fractures that Gehrig never bothered to mention. His streak of 2,130 consecutive games set a work standard not equaled until Cal Ripken Jr. passed that mark in 1995—a Gibraltar in cleats indeed.

Gehrig suffered from an illness that was unknown at the time—later diagnosed as ALS (amyotrophic lateral sclerosis), or more commonly, Lou Gehrig's disease. Gehrig persevered in the face of declining health, not knowing the cause or whether he would ever recover. At the beginning of the 1939 spring training season, Gehrig was simply not his old self, yet he carried on. He had not missed a game in over 2,100 appearances. On May 2 of that year, Gehrig told the Yankee manager, before what would be his 2,131st game, that he was benching himself "for the good of the team" and took himself off the lineup card, shocking the fans and his teammates, and ending his consecutive game streak at 2,130 (this record would stand until Cal Ripken, Jr., on September 6, 1995—tied the record that many thought was unbreakable. Ripken would later go on to amass a record of 2,632 consecutive games).

What is remarkable about Gehrig is that, despite this illness that eventually claimed his short life just seventeen days shy of his thirty-eighth birthday, he remained positive, focused, and embodied a level of courage and perseverance that has become a model for anyone who is privileged to wear the Yankee uniform. Gehrig was and is an icon of all that is good in baseball and in life.

Fans remember his farewell speech, but it is the picture of him on the day he told manager Joe McCarthy, "I'm benching myself, Joe," that embodies the ideal of perseverance. Gehrig is seen reclining against the dugout steps with a stoic expression on his face. It was May 2, 1939, and he knew he would never play the game he loved again.

# 12
# The Singing Bat

## The role of musical acoustics in baseball

Imagine if–from 350 feet away–you could recognize whether a ball is heading for the left-field bleachers or for a loop single to right–all from listening and paying attention to the repertoire of songs that baseball bats sing. Yes, you heard that right. Baseball bats can sing–and they all sing in different ways–some sing like Pavarotti while others sound like a bad contestant on *American Idol.* How do you tell the difference? Acoustics.

Acoustics are at the heart of great music. A well-designed concert hall–like Carnegie Hall in New York or Disney Concert Hall in Los Angeles–has amazing acoustics that allow the performers (and the audience) to hear music with a level of clarity that would otherwise be muddied in a less stellar concert hall.

Great musicians understand acoustics to a high level–they've developed a heightened sense of hearing, through years of studying and listening, which enables them to discern sounds and pitches. The sound of a fretless bass in the hands of a great jazz bassist–like a Jaco Pastorius–sounds acoustically different from that same electric bass in the hands of someone else.

Often times we recognize music not just through the melody, but the acoustics–the sounds and timbre–that musical instruments make. If you're listening to an obscure Beatles song on the radio that you've never heard before–you still recognize that it's the Beatles–solely from the sound, acoustics, and timbre.

Timbre in music is what distinguishes two notes of the same pitch and volume–like the difference in sound between an acoustic and an electric guitar playing the same note. The acoustics and timbre collectively create an audible roadmap that enables musicians to create a unique sound–like the Beatles.

But here is where it gets interesting: if you can train your ears to discern the differences in musical "timbre," those same ears can also be used to discern the differences in "timber"—as in the sound that a wood bat makes when it comes into contact with a baseball. In fact, you likely know what a home run sounds like. *Crack!*

Melvin Mora, who used to play for the Baltimore Orioles, could follow a ball simply by the acoustics and sound of the bat.

"As soon as I hear the sound of the bat, I know where the ball is going."

If it's a sharp crack, he races out—a dull clunk, and he runs in.

"It's about reaction," he said.

When pressed further, Mora replied, "It's something I can't explain."

But scientists have made it their business to understand one of the most unique relationships between music and baseball: sound.

Every bat is like a musical instrument—that when hit with a ball, sings in a different way. Scientists have studied the complex dynamics of wood bats when they smack a fastball, and have discovered that bats sing differently depending on whether the batter connects on a long drive or a weak fly ball. Physicists have also analyzed the ways in which players rely on and react to those sounds.

Any study of baseball acoustics was often relegated to stadium design, with an ear towards giving fans an unparalleled auditory experience that rivaled a rock concert. The first public-address system wasn't installed until 1929—in the Polo Grounds in New York. Now acousticians designing new ballparks are studying not only the acoustics of broadcasting sound over a large PA system, but how a ballpark's sounds can enhance the experience for players as well.

The crack of the bat when a home run is hit has a distinct, almost piercing sound to it. You can hear it on radio and in the last row of the bleachers. Dr. Robert Adair, a Yale physicist, who has studied the acoustics of bats hitting baseballs, says, "The crack of a well-hit ball is not just louder or sharper than the clunk of a ball hit off the end of the bat or off its handle, but a different sound completely." He went on to say that "A bat vibrates much like a guitar string, resonating with waves too slight for the eye to see. But those vibrations, involving frequencies of around 170 oscillations per second and higher, are what sting the hands of the batter who does not hit the ball solidly—and they generate the dull thud that starts outfielders running in."

"By contrast," he said, "a crack is the explosive sound of outrushing air when, for less than a millisecond, or thousandth of a second, the ball is clobbered so hard that it flattens and wraps itself fleetingly around the front of the bat.

"Although the ball always deforms a bit on contact, the effect is slight unless it makes a powerful and almost direct collision with the bat's 'sweet spot.' Most of the bat flexes and vibrates in wave motion when struck, but hitting the sweet spot is something like dropping a heavy rubber ball on the fulcrum of a seesaw: only at that point will the ball bounce back strongly rather than tipping the seesaw. Those stationary parts of the wave motion are called 'nodes.'

"If it's a crack, you know the ball is hit pretty hard, and you'd better start running backward,'" Dr. Adair says. "The eye simply cannot distinguish a bloop from a blast hit straight toward an outfielder for about the first 1.5 seconds of its flight," Dr. Adair said, referring to a separate calculation. "So acoustics and other clues are crucial."

Mora estimated that the jump he got from the sound alone—a crack or a clunk—amounts to about a step—which in baseball is a potential game changer. But when a monster home run is hit, the crack of the bat has such a distinctive and ominous sound that everyone in the stadium intuitively knows it.

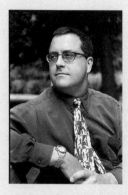

## VLADIMIR GUERRERO IN CONCERT

by Tim Wiles, baseball researcher and author, Cooperstown, New York

I was at Olympic Stadium in Montreal well before a game. Vladimir Guerrero was playing with the Montreal Expos back then and was taking batting practice all by himself. The stadium was empty, except for Guerrero, the pitcher, and me. The retractable roof was closed, which created a huge echo. It was a surreal sight to behold–an empty cavern, with only a few people inside–and there is Guerrero in the batter's box, pummeling home run after home run into the bleachers.

You'd hear this frightening, echoic *CRACK* followed by the whooshing sound of the ball breaking the air as it headed out into the stands. The "whoosh" echoed in a circular path around the inside of the stadium like a Tasmanian devil. Then came a deep, thunderous *THUD*–like a bomb dropping–as the ball hit the concrete, followed by a syncopated rhythm of *thud!–thud!–thud-thud-thud* as the ball careened and bounced over the seats.

With each *thud*, the ball would kick up a half-dozen or so panicked pigeons in different parts of the bleachers–wings flapping wildly, accompanied by screechy cooing that sounded like nails on a chalkboard. It was an amazing experience and I'll never forget the sounds. Guerrero put on quite a concert!

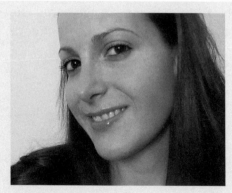

## TRAINING THE BRAIN

by Dr. Meagan Curtis, Ph.D., professor of psychology and lifelong Boston Red Sox fan

How do you get to Yankee Stadium? The same way you get to Carnegie Hall: practice, practice, practice! Acquiring expertise involves years of intense, daily practice. Malcolm Gladwell has estimated that it takes 10,000 hours of practice to become an expert (which is no small investment of time—if you practice four hours a day, 365 days a year, it would take you almost seven years to reach 10,000 hours of practice).

A mere hour of practice often produces measureable improvements; a pianist who struggles to get through a difficult passage may, after an hour of practice, be able to execute the passage perfectly. Within 10,000 hours of practice, a pianist may go from playing "Chopsticks" to playing Rachmaninoff's Piano Concerto No. 3. Within 10,000 hours of practice, a baseball player may go from playing Little League to being drafted by a major league franchise.

The effects of long-term practice on performance are profound. But how does this intense, long-term training influence the brain? Recent neuro-imaging evidence has shown that these years of training actually change the brain. The brains of musicians exhibit growth in areas of the motor cortex needed for executing the motor movements involved in playing instruments.

Growth has also been exhibited in the areas of the auditory cortex responsible for pitch perception, and the level of brain activation in response to pitch is also higher in musicians than in non-musicians. Although these changes in the auditory cortex are caused by musical training, they benefit the auditory perception of many types of sounds—even the sounds of baseball.

For instance, the characteristic crack of a bat striking a ball actually sounds different depending on which area of the barrel hits the ball. If a fielder uses the different barrel sounds to assess where the ball is likely to go, he will get a good jump on the ball and be more likely to make the play. A ballplayer who has developed his auditory cortex through musical training should be better at perceiving the different sounds of the bat.

Bernie's musical training may have directly contributed to his ability to process those bat sounds and get a jump on the ball; when we consider the fact that Bernie won four Golden Glove Awards, this seemingly small auditory-processing advantage may have yielded large performance gains. Musical training could potentially influence athletic performance in other ways as well. The corpus callosum, which allows the two hemispheres of the brain to communicate, is thicker in musicians, enhancing the motor coordination of the right and left sides of the body. Professional athletes obviously need to have excellent motor coordination, and it's possible that these musical enhancements may benefit athletic performance.

# 13
# The Art of Performing

How to develop your performance level

In order to perform at a high level–to be "in the zone"–you have to incorporate elements of real-life performance situations, whether on the field or on the stage. Ballplayers have it easier in this regard: from a young age, most young ballplayers spend considerable time playing the game–and by analogy, Little Leaguers in effect start playing concerts at the same time they're practicing their instruments, learning to play. High school ballplayers will play an average of twenty to forty (or more) games during a single season. And of course, in the major leagues, playing 162 games is analogous to a rock band being on tour performing nearly every other night for a year.

Younger, less experienced musicians, however, have it different. They'll spend the majority of their time practicing, and very little of it actually performing. Think about it: a typical student in high school, who practices one hour a day, might only have one school concert a semester. For every 100 hours of practicing, less than one hour is dedicated to performing.

For baseball players and musicians, nothing can replace the experience of playing in a real-life situation, whether it's performing on the field or on the stage. Even if you don't have the luxury of playing games or concerts on a regular basis, it's vital that you find opportunities to create performance situations and scenarios that test your ability to synthesize everything you've learned and apply it to the art of performance.

Performing–or playing the game–requires an entirely different psyche and mindset than practicing, and it is only through constant practice "performing" that any young musician or ballplayer can progress to the point where playing before a packed crowd–regardless of whether it's a ball game or a concert–will feel natural. You can be the greatest athlete or musician during practice, but if you can't translate your ability and apply it to a performance situation, then it doesn't matter how good you are during those practice situations. You could practice every waking hour of the day for ten years, but if you don't acquire the confidence to utilize what you practice in a performance situation, then it really doesn't matter what and how much you practice.

We are all built differently in terms of how we react in performance situations. Some younger musicians and ballplayers struggle with performing live in front of people. Young musicians, especially, can find the experience so foreign and fraught with anxiety that they shy away from it. Getting through this stage in your development as a "performer" is paramount. It's not something to avoid.

The first step in transitioning from a practice situation to a live performance situation is to be thoroughly prepared. If you're at bat or onstage and you're not prepared, your experience is likely to be less than stellar. It's only through thorough preparation that you'll gain the confidence you need to deliver a great performance.

The second step is to be able to focus and override the anxiety, nervousness, and the crowd or audience. Walking onstage or walking to the plate for the first time can be a traumatic experience if you're not able to focus. As any great ballplayer or musician will tell you, there is nothing that prepares you entirely for that moment of stepping out and being greeted by a stadium or arena packed with screaming fans. If ever there is a place or time to lose your focus, this is likely it. But you can't. You need to be strong in your mind and your approach.

The third step is crucial: you need to block out any analytical or critical thoughts from your mind. All the fundamentals and mechanics that you honed through hours of diligent practice and study–the muscle memory that you've acquired–now need to subside into the background and be totally off your radar in a performance situation. The first time onstage or in a pressure situation on the field might leave you filled with anxiety and butterflies in your stomach. Understand that the true reason that you are nervous is that the situation you are in is–first and foremost–simply unfamiliar to you, which leads you to have doubts and thoughts of failing.

This is a scenario which many a young ballplayer and musician face early on, and it is important to embrace it–to run through it–so that you get to the other side of it, where you are in control, relaxed, and at peace. There is no shame in failing in performance, especially if you have prepared well. In fact, it is through failing that we learn to become more comfortable with performing in a high-pressure situation. In other words, the fear of failure, the anxiety, and the nervousness eventually become familiar to us–and once they become familiar and commonplace, these feelings will start to dissipate, replaced by confidence.

The fourth step involves ensuring that your level of preparation is appropriate to the performance situation. As vital as practice and preparation are, there is danger in over-preparing for a performance if it supersedes the actual performance. It can't take away anything that you must reserve for the performance. Many players can get so involved with practice and preparation that at the time of the game or concert, they are not at their best because they are physically and or mentally tired. You have to realize that the two to three hours you spend onstage or on the field cannot be usurped by your practice, especially the day of the performance.

## FEAR OF SUCCESS

by Bernie Williams

When you've had a great performance–a breakout moment on the field or on the stage–you might be tempted to doubt whether you can repeat it and doubt that you can consistently perform at that level. It's important that you don't treat these moments as flukes.

Willie Randolph once said to me, "Bernie, don't be afraid of success–people get afraid because they think they'll now have to maintain that level, and suddenly, there's pressure on them. Just assume that this is the way you do business." He was right—accept those breakout moments. Don't put added pressure on yourself and think, "How am I going to do this every time I'm onstage or at bat?" Instead, just focus on doing what you've been doing, and let the results be what they may.

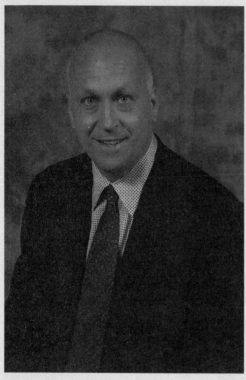

# SECOND NATURE

..................................

by Cal Ripken, Jr., Baseball Hall of Famer, 2007

..................................

My dad used to have a saying, "Practice doesn't make perfect—perfect practice makes perfect." Now, a lot of people who heard that took it to mean that you couldn't make mistakes in practice—that it wasn't fun—things like that. What Dad meant was simply that when you are practicing and preparing to compete, you should go through the drills the same way you would in a game. It is impossible to flip a switch and improve things if you aren't doing it correctly during practice. Practice is the time to try things differently and experiment, but once you determine the best way to do something, practice it that way over and over again so when it is time to do it in the game—or concert—it will be second nature.

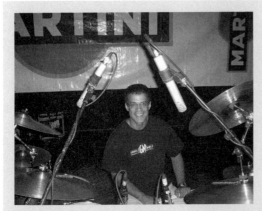

## GROOVE CATCHER

Richie Morales, drummer with Bernie Williams, Spyro Gyra, Mike Stern, Grover Washington, Jr., the Brecker Brothers, two generations of Brubecks, and others

A drummer is like a catcher on the field, controlling the inning, calling the pitches, and managing the game—saying, "Go with me, guys," and creating the groove that enables the other players to perform well. A great pitching-catching duo is like a good jazz drummer backing up the soloist, providing the foundation for the soloist to shine. A certain amount of trust needs to exist—if the pitcher keeps shaking the catcher off, sooner or later, he's gonna get one jacked out of the park. A truly great musician or ballplayer elevates the level of performance of everyone around them.

Remember not to allow preparation to supersede or jeopardize the quality of a performance. Performance is about being and executing in the moment. I remember being on tour with Dave Brubeck, and his drummer, the legendary Alan Dawson, would warm up religiously before the gig—then stop at a certain point and say, "That's enough—I don't want to leave it all here in the dressing room." And remember above all to have fun. I was in a rehearsal once with the great guitarist Hiram Bullock. At one point, things got a little tense, Hiram stopped and said, "You know, man, it's music—it's not nuclear war!"

## NINE THOUGHT ZONES

by Don Greene

There is a wide range of different types of performance thoughts in music and sports. They can be placed on a scale from 1 to 9. The nine mental performance zones range from the most damaging thoughts to peak-performance thoughts.

1. The most damaging thoughts are the fear-based, negative-outcome thoughts, and helplessness. Examples of these include: "I'm afraid of losing"; "It would be devastating if I failed"; "You won't be able to handle it"; "This is not going to go well"; "It's impossible"; and "I'm probably going to choke." Such fearful thoughts focus on the worst happening and cause anxiety, distraction, and muscle tension.

2. The second type of thought, slightly less damaging, includes doubts, self-criticism, and blaming. Examples of these thoughts include: "I don't think I can do this"; "I'm not so sure if I have the ability"; "I should have prepared better beforehand." During the performance, it may be: "This isn't very good"; "Can't you do any better than that?"; and "I suck." Afterwards, it may be: "I wish I had a good teacher" or "I need to find a better accompanist."

3. The third type of thought is counterproductive to optimal performance. These include frustration, negative perceptions, and wrong interpretations. Examples of frustrated thinking are: "I still can't do this"; "It's taking forever"; and "I'll never be able to do this damn thing." Negative perceptions include: "I don't feel comfortable here"; "I'm nervous"; or "This is not a good time for me." It can also include neutral circumstances—like seeing a traffic accident en route to a performance—as an omen or bad sign: "It means that I'm not going to do well"; "Maybe I should cancel"; or "I don't want to have a disaster like that."

4. The fourth type is unhelpful thoughts. These include outcome thoughts, unnecessary instructions, and meaningless feedback. Examples of outcome thoughts are: "You've got to win this time"; "It may be your last chance"; or "It's now or never." Instructions, like "You can't make any mistakes" and "It's got to be perfect," don't help performers under pressure. Verbal feedback, like "You're not doing very well" or "This doesn't sound very good," are also unhelpful.

5. The next type is unnecessary thought. These include thoughts about others' opinions, ongoing commentary, and boredom. The first pertains to what others are thinking about one's performance: "Do they like my style?"; "Do they think I'm any good?"; or "They don't think I'm very good." Examples of other unnecessary thoughts: "I guess it's going alright"; "It doesn't sound all that bad"; and "I wish I was into it more; it's just not very important."

6. The sixth type of thought is helpful for performers. These helpful thoughts include positive perceptions, correct interpretations, and discernment. The

positive perceptions are thoughts such as: "I'm feeling really energized"; "I'm really psyched up to do my best"; and "The adrenaline's starting to kick in." An example of interpreting neutral circumstances correctly is: "That means I'm going to do well." Discernment, rather than judgment, is also helpful: "You're slightly sharp" or "I'm behind the beat."

7. The seventh type is functional thought. This includes necessary adjustments, process thinking, and confident thoughts. Following discernment, the adjustments are straightforward: "Get back on pitch" or "Pick up the right tempo." Process thinking is related to correct execution, like "Keep in balance" or "Stay with it." Examples of confident thoughts are: "I can do this"; "I'm really good at this"; and "I know I can do well this time."

8. The next type of performance thought is optimal thinking. These thoughts are based in imagination, optimism, and courage. The imagined thoughts are about how the performance would go well, how it would look, sound, and feel. Optimal thinking would also include: "I think it's going to be great" and "I know I'm ready to do my best." A good example of courageous thought: "Go for it!"

9. The ninth type is peak-performance thinking. This includes thoughts of empowerment ("I can do anything I set my mind to"), focus ("Center"), freedom ("Let it fly!"), love, joy, and gratitude. Other than the mental quiet of alpha, these types of thoughts are the best by far.

Here's an exercise I used in my Juilliard class. I told the students that they were to set up a performance situation. After warming up, they were to put three mid-difficulty excerpts from their repertoire on a music stand in a practice room. Before leaving the room, they were to place their instrument in a handy place and turn a tape recorder on in the room. They were then to leave the room, go up and down three flights of stairs, pause briefly outside the room, and then enter the room.

Once they picked up their instrument and got set, they were to perform the three pieces back to back without stopping. After they were finished and turned the tape recorder off, I asked them to identify their predominant type of thinking during each of the pieces.

The students were to repeat the exercise until they were consistently performing with positive thoughts, or none at all. Then they were to listen to the first recording and the latest recordings and compare them. By the next class, most of the students really got it and heard the dramatic difference in the quality of their sound. After a few weeks, their teachers started to hear it too.

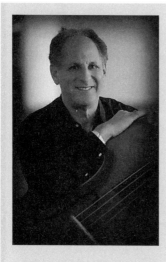

# P=P-I

by Barry Green, author of *The Inner Game of Music*

The basic truth is that our performance of any task depends as much on the extent to which we interfere with our abilities as it does on those abilities themselves. This can be expressed as a formula:

$$P = p - i$$

In this equation, *P* refers to *performance*, which we define as the result you achieve–what you actually wind up feeling, achieving, and learning. Similarly, *p* stands for *potential*, defined as your innate ability–what you are naturally capable of. And *i* means *interference*–your capacity to get in your own way.

# 14
# The Art of the Reboot

## The psychology of the slump

*Nearly every man who develops an idea works at it up to the point where it looks impossible, and then gets discouraged. That's not the place to become discouraged.*
–THOMAS EDISON

*This too shall pass.*
–ANCIENT PERSIAN PROVERB

I've been through slumps! The worst one was at the beginning of the 1994 season, when I was only hitting .168 through May 9. I hit four home runs and had eleven RBIs, but I also went through two 0-for-11 streaks and one of 0-for-18. It was one of the toughest times in my career.

But I broke out of it–and hit .326 for the rest of the season. Slumps don't last forever.

There comes a time in every musician's or athlete's career when all your hard work and effort don't produce the results you want and nothing seems to be going right. In baseball, it's called the dreaded "slump"–and it can be extremely frustrating to experience psychologically, mentally, and emotionally. Going through a slump is a bit of a mystery too–often times, nothing seems to help and you're likely perplexed as to why you're not making progress.

Slumps are the bane of a ballplayer's existence. They come out of nowhere, outstay their welcome, and ironically, leave when we least expect them to. Slumps take us out of the zone and make it difficult to focus. Our mind starts to play tricks on us, spreading the seeds of self-doubt.

During a slump, you're not able to process everything the way you normally do—during an at bat, you may feel rushed, and your brain is not able to process the information accordingly. Your perception is skewed, and you can't tell with enough clarity what the ball's location and rotation is, your mind and body are out of sync, and you feel sluggish. If you're playing defense, you might rush catching the ball, not paying attention to the position of your glove, and the ball bounces out. Instead of everything slowing down, everything starts to speed up!

The truth is that all great players and musicians experience peaks and valleys, ups and downs. It's a fact of life, and the sooner you can accept it as a part of being human, the better off you'll be. However, it's the great players who know how to minimize the time spent in these slumps. The biggest factor in minimizing slumps is maintaining a positive attitude and self-confidence. Slumps are no more unnatural than breathing—we're not robots, and our bodies and minds simply cannot operate at peak efficiency all the time. Great players understand this—and have the ability to bounce right back.

Slumps are roughly 80 percent psychological and 20 percent physical, and usually begin with a mental breakdown first, in which a player experiences doubt or insecurity. Maybe they struck out three times in the last game, and it starts to weigh in on them. Perhaps they're unintentionally trying to out-think themselves, or paying too much attention to results rather than their approach. Perhaps a player is trying to improve too much too quickly, seeking advice from too many places, and all this new information is cluttering their mind.

It's at this point that a player will start to tinker with their mechanics, which is precisely what you don't want to be doing early on in a slump. Once you start second-guessing your basic mechanics, you'll be inclined to overcompensate. Perhaps because of those three strikeouts, you'll start to hurry your swing, which paradoxically will cause your bat speed to decrease! It is very important at this early point in a slump not to overreact, or the next thing you know—you're hitless in your last twenty-five at bats!

What is crucial in slumps is that you remain hyper-focused and in tune with your body. Don't change anything that was working fine before the slump began. Watch videos of your swing and consult with your coaches. A good coach can teach you new things–but a great coach can detect faults in your mechanics. Remember: you can't solve a problem if you don't know first exactly what the problem is.

You also need to stay strong physically and continue to develop your strength and endurance so that you don't become complacent with your mechanics. Some players, early on in slumps, will forsake their routine too soon, and this can be a catalyst for prolonging the slump, snowballing the player into a much more protracted slump than they would have had if they had stuck with their physical routine and conditioning.

There are several key steps to take in addressing prolonged slumps, and several important things to know. The first thing to know is that slumps are inevitable–they are as much a part of the rhythms of life as they are a part of the rhythms of the game. Obviously, we all want to minimize the length of a slump. Second, slumps should be accepted for what they are–temporary. There exists no great musician or ballplayer who didn't experience a slump of some kind. Embrace it with a positive attitude, and above all, learn from it. It could be that the slump is telling you something. It could also be that you're body is simply mentally, physically, or emotionally fatigued. Whatever the reasons for a prolonged slump, the fact is that you're not likely to break out of it as soon as you can unless you do the following: shut down.

When all else fails, and players are in a long protracted slump where nothing seems to work, it's time to "shut down" everything and reboot. In shutdown mode, it's like pushing a reset button, rebooting yourself, both in mind and body. Sometimes, in order to reboot, you have to drastically change your daily routine and schedule, the exact opposite of what you would want to do early on in a slump.

Perhaps you're always up at 6:00 a.m.? Sleep in late! If

you're practicing all day, take a day off. Do things that break your routine and get your mind off of what is frustrating you. Go to a ball game (if you're a musician) or a concert (if you're a ballplayer). Above all, it's important to change your routine.

During this "reboot" phase, abandon all your preconceptions of how you approach your craft. Return to the building blocks and review your fundamentals. Try different approaches and different angles. Experiment. Seek out advice and try something new. The amount of time you spend in this phase is dependent, more than most players realize, on maintaining perspective and a positive attitude. There is absolutely no substitute for these two qualities for a player in the midst of a protracted slump.

Breaking out of a slump is a mystery. It just happens when you least expect it. You could be having a terrible day, feeling awful, and suddenly–you're at bat, trying to figure out a pitcher, you foul a ball back–and something just clicks. In that moment, something profound is revealed and you say to yourself, "I got it!" The pitcher looks at you differently because he sees your demeanor change in that one foul ball. It's a mystery. It's magic. And then you start to laugh at that slump–all the things that caused you to get into that slump now seem meaningless and innocuous. It's over–you know it, your teammates know it, and the other team knows it. It's a wonderful feeling–the clouds part, the rain stops, and life goes on. You feel lighter, the pressure's off, and a great burden has been mysteriously lifted from your shoulders. You feel grateful, thankful, and the game becomes fun again.

# CENTERING

by Don Greene

When you're in a protracted slump and need to reboot, the centering process can be enormously helpful. Centering is a focusing strategy based on principles from the Japanese martial art of aikido, specific breathing techniques, and different ways to access the right-brain alpha state. Centering has repeatedly proven to significantly improve the performance of competitive athletes and elite musicians performing under pressure. Furthermore, after practice and mastering the technique, centering can be done anywhere, sitting or standing, in less than ten seconds.

To try the long form of centering, find a comfortable sitting position with your back straight. Have your hands over your center, located two inches below your navel and two inches into your body. Make sure that you feel in balance.

Step 1. Direct your eyes to your focus point. This is a precise spot about 1–20 feet in front of you, but always below eye level. If your eyes go up, you go into left-brain thinking. It's easier to access the right brain and alpha with your eyes down or closed.

Step 2. Say, "Now I am going to center," to yourself.

Step 3. Close your eyes or soften your focus (daydream in the direction of the floor). Breathe in slowly through your nose to a count of seven, pause for a count of seven, and then breathe slowly out through your mouth for a count of seven. Pull each breath in as deep and as low as possible through your nose, pause and hold it, and then exhale slowly out through your mouth. Take seven or more breaths, until you're focused only on your breathing.

Step 4. Continuing to breath that way, scan your upper body for muscle tension. Breathe in slowly and deeply through your nose and notice if your jaw feels tight. Pause and feel free to move it around. Then breathe out whatever tension you may find there. Then breathe in and check to see if your neck feels tight. Pause and then release the tension as you breathe out. Then check your shoulders and let go of any tightness you find as you breathe out. Then check your arms and hand, and breath out the tension.

Step 5. Breathe slowly and deeply into your center, pause, and then breathe out. Breathe in slowly, focus on your center, breath out. Take seven or more breaths until you feel that you're at your center.

Step 6. Clearly hear the sound you'd like to produce, watch the mental movie of how you'd love to perform, or feel the movement you'd like to create.

Step 7. After forming the desired sound, image, or feeling in your right brain, direct your eyes back to your focus point and say, "Now I'm centered and ready to go."

When you start practicing centering, it should take you one to three minutes. Your ability to center will improve with correct practice and repetition. You can start out by practicing the long form of the centering process three to seven times a day. If you use it as part of your normal routine, before you warm up, practice, or perform, you will notice positive effects within a few weeks. Eventually, with practice, you will be able to do the advanced form of centering, which takes ten seconds or less.

The goal for now is not to see how fast you can do it, but to accomplish the task of each step in the centering process. Find a balanced position. Make sure that you pick your focus point and say, "Now I'm going to center." Then focus on your breathing before scanning your muscles for tension. Take as many breaths as you need. Find your center and then be there. Hear the sound you'd like to produce, the way you want it to look, or the feeling you intend to experience. Then with your eyes on the focal point, say, "Now I'm centered and ready to go."

# PLAYING WITH PAIN

by Dave Gluck

Baseball fans might be surprised to learn that musicians suffer from injury as much as ballplayers. Tendonitis, carpel-tunnel syndrome, and bursitis are just some of the injuries that musicians face. We may not be pulling quads or hamstrings, but we can experience debilitating pain in our arms, neck, hands, and shoulders to the point where we're unable to play. Many of these injuries are a result of repetitive strain and overuse while other injuries can be traced to poor posture. There's a fourth category, though, and I wasn't aware of it until, by accident, my Tai Chi instructor pointed it out.

I had acquired an acute case of bursitis in my right shoulder, which was causing me a lot of pain. Being a professional drummer, the pain was so debilitating that it placed my career in jeopardy. I tried everything—massage therapy, chiropractic sessions, acupuncture, etc.—but nothing worked. I was in a Tai Chi class one day and mentioned the pain to my instructor. She asked if she could observe me while practicing on a drum set.

For about twenty minutes, all she did was sit and observe. And then she got up while I was playing and gently applied pressure to my shoulder with her finger. The pain seared through my shoulder and down my spine. Her finger felt like a chisel going through my shoulder, and I winced. "Something's not right," she said. She pointed to my ride cymbal that I was playing with my right hand. "Can you lower it a quarter inch?" I began to doubt she could help—after all, a quarter inch isn't such a big difference, right?

Within thirty minutes, the pain had subsided. I was dumbfounded. She saw something that only an expert in Tai Chi could see—that by having that ride cymbal a fraction of an inch too high, I was placing unnecessary strain on my body. My movements and posture weren't natural, all because of that quarter of an inch. It was through this experience that I discovered the importance of playing ergonomically. Ergonomics can have a huge impact on a musician's life. Holding a drumstick, a guitar, or a trumpet in your hand for four to six hours a day can wreak havoc on your natural body movement if the instrument and you are not postured in a way that is natural.

It's vital that your instrument becomes a natural extension of your body, and that it accommodates your natural movements. This is particularly important when you play an instrument like a drum set, which has several different components. It's also critical that you develop a constant awareness of your body's relationship to your instrument, just like a hitter with a bat, a pitcher with a ball, and a fielder with a glove.

Bad habits occur when you're not fully aware of your body and its movements. Tension can creep in, flaws start to develop, and you can end up in a slump, just like a hitter. This is why rudiments and basics are so critical to both musicians and ballplayers—they keep us in touch with our body, ensuring that our movements and mechanics are efficient, relaxed, and correct.

# KEEPING TIME

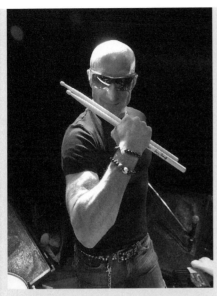

by Kenny Aronoff, drummer with Bernie Williams, the Smashing Pumpkins, John Mellencamp, Jon Bon Jovi, Elton John, Puddle of Mudd, and many others

Great ballplayers and great musicians share this in common: they know what it takes to push themselves far beyond what is normal. The best musicians take care of themselves. Despite what you may have heard about the life of rock musicians, the reality is that my entire day revolves around what I eat, the vitamins I take, and what kind of exercise I do. I try to drink a gallon of water each day and eat healthy.

There are three things that I find in common among musicians and baseball players—a hard work ethic, a willingness to learn and relearn, and finally passion. This is what fuels hard work—the desire to be great. My advice to young musicians and ballplayers is this: outgrow doubt. You have to accept the human condition that we all make mistakes—things go wrong that are out of your control. You have to accept it, adapt to it, and move on. Never give up—focus on being the best that you can be. Remember, you can't hurry experience—you can't get it all as a kid.

My mantra in music and life is this: I'll never be as great as I want to be—but I'll spend the rest of my life trying to be the best that I can be.

# 15
# Batting Practice

A creative approach to practicing
fundamentals

Before and after every game I played with the New York Yankees, I worked diligently on the basics and fundamentals of the game. In order to excel at music or baseball, a significant portion of your daily routine has to center on the fundamentals and the basics.

Part of the reason for focusing on the most rudimentary aspects of either music or baseball is simply to slow things down. You can't get any slower than playing a long tone on your instrument or simply hitting a ball off of a tee–and if you can't correctly hit a stationary ball off of a tee, there is certainly no way you'll be able to consistently hit one thrown to you.

Slowing things down also allows us to identify and isolate bad habits we may have unconsciously acquired. Bad technique and habits form when we're not diligent and forget to focus on whether our mechanics and fundamentals are in order. We're not machines–we're human beings that are in a state of continual change, growth, and renewal. We have good days and bad days, we get tired, and there are a myriad of influences that shape how we move and think.

Musicians, no matter how advanced they may be, often spend hours per week working on and repeating the most simple and basic exercises. Why? To ensure that their mechanics are solid and that their muscle memory is properly tuned to a point where they don't have to think about it when they're on the stage. When you're at bat, you don't want to be focusing on your mechanics, using your analytical left brain–you want to be in the zone, using your right brain to think intuitively, creatively, and artistically. Developing muscle memory affects the quickness and accuracy of your reflexes. If your muscle memory isn't developed properly, you'll either miss that note or miss the ball.

Another important part of basic exercises is simply to allow the body to warm up properly. The human body contains more than 650 skeletal muscles that affect our strength, balance, posture, and movement. The two main causes of injury among musicians and athletes are overuse of certain muscles (i.e., when a pitcher's arm is injured from simply pitching too much) or not having enough elasticity (as when a runner pulls a quad muscle or a tendon). What you'll find among great ballplayers and musicians is acute attention to fundamentals. No great athlete or musician ignores them in their daily routine. It is the lifeblood of what we do.

Great players have honed their mechanics and basics to such a high level that they're able to focus creatively on the game, making intuitive, game-altering decisions before their left brain even has time to catch up to what has happened. The more important point, though, is that—before you can allow the more intuitive and creative right side of your brain to take control of the helm when making and responding to situations, the more analytical and critical-thinking left side of your brain has to crystallize the raw material (the muscle memory you learn from practicing the fundamentals) so that it can eventually be used artistically.

So much of baseball—and music as well—is based on reflexive decision-making. There's no time to consciously think about it: your body and mind simply have to react. It is only through constant repetition that your mind and body can reflexively start to recognize pitches and their location. For instance, a ninety-five-mile-an-hour pitch simply doesn't allow the brain time to consciously process enough information to respond accordingly. It is only through muscle memory—hitting enough ninety-five-mile-an-hour fastballs—that your eyes, brain, and muscles start to develop a level of coordination that can be memorized intuitively. In a split second, the eyes see the ball, which your brain interprets as–let's say, an inside fastball–sending a message to your body to swing. If you have to think about hitting a fastball in the mid-nineties, you've already swung and missed.

Young players often try to learn the fundamentals of hitting and fielding from watching their favorite major league players. There is a lot to be learned from watching great players, to be sure–but where it's not helpful is trying to imitate or mimic those players. No two players are the same, and the batting stance that works for a Jorge Posada may not work for a Derek Jeter. Everyone is built differently, and some players at the major league level develop a very personalized approach to hitting and fielding that works for them and only them.

Rather than trying to imitate great players, focus on the mechanics of those players and try to simplify your approach, such that your basic mechanics are all working as they should. When you're up at bat, be sure your head, legs, and arms are all relaxed and properly positioned and their weight properly distributed. No matter what the batting stance, great players are all relaxed when they come to the plate, and while some may have an unorthodox swing or stance that works for them, it could spell disaster for the young player trying to imitate it. The game of baseball is complicated enough–don't make it even more complicated by trying to circumvent good mechanics in favor of swinging away like the major league player you saw hit that grand slam the night before!

This is not to say that there aren't variations within good mechanics–there are. In some instances, there are no right or wrong ways of doing certain things–there can even be a certain amount of variables within basic mechanics. But for younger players, focus first on developing solid, good mechanics. Once you've mastered this, you can progress to find your own variation on a swing. By practicing the fundamentals daily and developing good, solid mechanics, we gain the confidence of knowing that we've covered every aspect of our game.

A good example of players focusing on their mechanics, and perhaps the most visible for baseball fans, is watching players take batting practice. Batting practice is a relaxing time—a time to slow things down and focus on the mechanics and basics of a good swing. With the Yankees, a complete batting practice session for me consisted of three phases, starting with phase one (hitting a stationary ball on a tee), progressing to phase two (hitting a ball slowly tossed underhand), and finally to phase three (batters being pitched to at a constant speed from the mound, which is what fans see at the ballpark). If things are working well for you and you're not in a slump, players will skip over phase one. However, during the off-season, it's not uncommon for a hitting coach (like Kevin Long of the Yankees) to have a player start with hitting off of a tee, especially if they've struggled a bit the previous season.

The entire purpose of a complete batting practice session is to slow things down to a point where you can analyze and control the variables. There is no guesswork involved—batters are being pitched the same pitch at the same speed over and over again, reducing all the variables to a constant that allows you to focus entirely on your mechanics so that you can analyze what you're doing right or wrong, and make adjustments to improve.

As you progress from phase one to phase three, the variables are increased. Within phase three, there can be many variations, progressing from a few variables to many. For example, a typical phase-three batting practice might be divided as follows:

Round 1: Bunts
Round 2: Hit and run (guaranteed contact)
Round 3: Hitting to the opposite field, pulling the ball, etc. (in order to move a runner over)
Round 4: Situational hitting (practicing every possible scenario—e.g., a runner is on third, there are no outs, and you have to bring him home)

Finally, when these three phases are complete, batters move on to free swinging, where they can apply all that they have learned or have been working on to simply hit away. The structure of free swinging is a little looser, but players are still trying to work within a realistic, game-like framework.

Ironically, the longest home run I ever hit didn't happen in a game–it happened during batting practice! It was July 22, 2001, and I was taking batting practice before a Toronto Blue Jays game and hit the ball out of Yankee Stadium. I sometimes used batting practice to get all my frustrations out, and I'd always hit the ball hard–you never really get to take a full hack in a real game–but that was the hardest I've ever hit a baseball.

Apart from getting out your frustrations, batting practice is also a time to have fun, relax, and socialize with your teammates–and even the opposing players. There is even something of a party atmosphere, and for the fans, it's pure entertainment watching balls arch up into the sky and disappear in the outfield seats. It's one of the purest rituals of the game.

# ALPHA BETA

by Don Greene

In an earlier chapter, titled "The Matrix Moment," Bernie talked about being in the alpha state while taking a high school biology exam–and hitting a home run in extra innings during the playoffs. Understanding alpha and beta is important when you're working on fundamentals and focusing on improving your performance level.

There are four main patterns, or frequencies, as measured on a biofeedback machine in cycles per second (cps). Delta is our deepest state of sleep (4–7 cps), just enough to keep the physical system going. Theta is the frequency of brainwave activity when we're dreaming in REM sleep (8–13 cps).

Alpha is the brainwave pattern of the creative state, hypnosis, quiet focus, and meditation (11–13 cps). This alpha state exists at the borderline between waking consciousness and the subconscious. Once in alpha, you have direct and immediate access to proactively programming the subconscious with whatever you would like to create or cause to happen in reality.

We often pass through the alpha state during reverie (just as we're drifting off into theta sleep), after a beer or glass of wine, and sometimes upon awakening. If you can, just lie there and relax for a few moments before opening your eyes and starting the day's to-do list. Not necessarily easy.

That's because in beta, the normal state of waking consciousness in our fast-paced and multitasking society. Beta is defined as anything greater than 14 cps. Beta is the frequency of rapid fire, left-brain thinking in words and numbers. It's encouraged in school. The classroom competition is often about who can raise their hands first with answers to verbal questions and solutions to math problems.

Beta is closely associated with the left brain. Although it can be somewhat helpful as a problem-solving device, the left brain overanalyzes and produces suboptimal performances. The higher the beta brainwave activity, the worse the athletic or musical performance gets. In extreme conditions, beta can get up to 40 cps and spin totally out of control.

Alpha brainwaves are associated more with the right brain and much better suited for optimal and peak performances in music and sports. Alpha waves are slower and quieter than the rapid and noisy beta–especially the higher beta states associated with panic, distraction, and confusion. Alpha is much better for clear and effective thinking and being able to focus and perform well under pressure. The ability to achieve alpha on command is vital for creating optimal and peak performances.

There are many ways to achieve the alpha state: mindful breathing, centering, guided imagery, creative visualization, meditation, prayer, biofeedback training, hypnosis, listening to music (especially Mozart), playing music (like jazz), mantras, Zen practices, tai chi, yoga, and baseball.

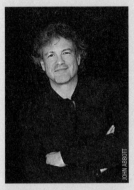

## BETWEEN THE EARS

by Pete Malinverni, jazz pianist, composer, and teacher, who has performed his original music at the Blue Note and Carnegie Hall

The most obvious parallel I see between baseball and music is that both the musician in performance and the ballplayer in a game are possessed of unquestioned gifts and hard-won skills, but are engaged in the attempt to achieve excellence in that one, most important, moment.

In the rehearsal room or practice field, you may have played that phrase or made the relay throw, beautifully struck that note or slyly waited on the curveball a thousand times before, but can you do it now with people watching and listening?

Ballplayers and musicians work hard over long years to master their arts, but the game and the music are played mostly between the ears—each of us must find that calm place wherein we can execute those things, impossible for the great majority of humans, that we've learned to do—and make them look easy.

The big difference, as I see it, is the fact that even when out of town, the musician rarely finds thousands rooting for him to fail. I have, however, had one or two beers spilled on me.

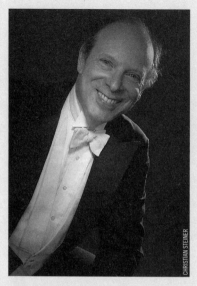

CHRISTIAN STEINER

# A STEINWAY IN CENTER FIELD

by Steven Lubin, concert pianist and classical recording artist

It may come as a surprise to fans of baseball that classical pianists are athletes as well. We need as much athleticism, strength, and endurance as major league ballplayers—in our hands. Two of the most demanding works for piano—Beethoven's "Emperor" Concerto and Rachmaninoff's Third Concerto—are each about forty minutes in duration. And you're at bat the entire time and you can't step out of the batter's box.

As a classical pianist playing this challenging repertoire, your degree of athleticism is utterly exposed—you're like an outfielder trying to run down a ball in the gap in front of thousands of fans. In order to play Beethoven's Waldstein Piano Sonata, one of his greatest works, I really have to tax and challenge my athleticism. It's a test of speed, strength, accuracy, and endurance.

Certainly, athleticism in music and baseball is all about what your body does in a particular situation—seemingly all by itself without a thought to guide it. In one of the most dramatic moments of my childhood, I remember playing center field—the game was tied in the late innings, with a kid on third and one out. I was playing pretty shallow—and then—*crack!* A fly ball's hit deep to right center. I sprinted flat out—caught the ball, planted my right foot, spun around, and fired home. The guy on third thought he would tag—but as soon as he saw my throw, he headed back to base. It may have been the best ten seconds of my life.

But on to the burning question: athleticism is fine, but is it art? Isn't artistry something quite separate from athleticism? After one concert, I was confronted by a concertgoer who was disappointed in my performance because she had paid for artistry but all she felt she got was athleticism.

"Why do you have to play like some sort of athlete in a stadium?" she asked indignantly. "Don't you think there might be other qualities in the music with which you could connect—like gentleness? Or how about humor?" Wow.

She believed that athleticism could never aspire to art—that the two are un-related and dissimilar, and that only art speaks directly to the soul, whereas athleticism appeals to the lower and shallower in us. I wanted to tell her to go see a great major league ball game—she might have seen that it's all one.

In my mind, artistry and athleticism are indistinguishably linked when it comes to execution. In music, athleticism is the skill required to make every-thing disappear except for the beauty of a composition's structural hierarchy. It's the skill of eliminating distractions—a skill that gives you control over your body to prevent inessential things from happening, like mistakes. In music, athleticism and technique are really the same thing.

Perhaps that's why I'm so proud of that fielding play I once made. There's a certain "supposed to" imbedded in a play like that. In a flash I'm supposed to run, catch the ball, fire a hard low throw to home, and save a run. For ten brief seconds in my childhood, my athleticism made everything irrelevant to the task disappear. It's exactly like what happens when I sit down to play Beethoven. Great athleticism is art, whether it's playing baseball or Beethoven. There will always be a space in my mind where the work of a pianist and ball-player converge. They're both about creating something beautiful—and mak-ing the irrelevant disappear.

# 16
# Snow on the Field

## What to do between tours and seasons

*It breaks your heart. It is designed to break your heart.*
*The game begins in the spring, when everything else begins again,*
*and it blossoms in the summer, filling the afternoons and evenings,*
*and then as soon as the chill rains come,*
*it stops and leaves you to face the fall alone.*
−BART GIAMATTI, "THE GREEN FIELDS OF THE MIND"

When the baseball season ends in October (and I always hoped it would end in October or November, and not earlier), you might think that professional baseball players get a vacation until spring training begins. Part of this is true–players get to finally spend extended time with their families and children. For both touring musicians and professional ballplayers, life on the road is grueling and tough–but the hardest part, especially for ballplayers and musicians with young children, is simply being away for upwards of seven–eight months from their families. You miss so much–the parent-teacher conferences, the recitals, dance performances, and so on. So the off-season is vital to the emotional well-being of ballplayers and musicians, their wives, and children.

It's not, however, a time to simply chill out in front of the television for four months. You have to remain healthy and in shape, lest you lose your agility and flexibility. I've found that any real growth, as a ballplayer or musician, has occurred off-season and when I'm not touring giving concerts. During the season, you're simply trying to maintain your level of performance–but it is in the off-season that you have the opportunity to improve so that next season (or the next tour) will bring greater success. As ballplayers get older, the off-season routine becomes more critical, and you have to work even harder to make those improvements.

There's basically three phases to the off-season for professional ballplayers. It starts almost immediately after the last game of the season with an active rest phase. During this phase, you engage in jogging, cardio workouts, etc. to keep your heart rate up. You never totally shut down your body during the off-season and it's vital to keep exercising for a month or so. The second phase is devoted to adding strength-training exercises. This is where you lift weights so that you can build up muscle mass in addition to continuing with cardio workouts. At the completion of these two phases, you need to be in top condition as a general athlete. During the off-season, pitchers will work on their repertoire of pitches, just like a musician would work on new songs for the next tour.

The off-season is critical for pitchers–this is where they can grow and add to the arsenal of pitches or refine the ones they already have. If you haven't used the off-season time wisely, by the time you get to spring training, you might be so far behind the curve that you'll spend a good part of the time catching up, beginning the season ill-prepared and start in a slump come April. The goal is to be so well prepared–mentally, physically, and emotionally–that when spring training starts, you can hit the ground running at full speed.

The third and final phase is, of course, spring training, that time-honored tradition where you spend late winter in Florida or Arizona, working together to develop team skills as well as on individual drills and exercises. The oddest part of spring training is putting on cleats for the first time after four months–you actually have to get used to wearing cleats again. Pitchers and catchers report a week earlier to spring training, and then the position players report, and the team for the next season is together for the first time.

There's an air of excitement and camaraderie. You haven't seen some of your teammates for four months (or longer if you're not in the postseason) and you catch up on how everybody is doing, trading stories and enjoying the feeling of being back together again in anticipation of the start of the new season.

Spring training is when you work on your muscle memory through repetition, and the structure of team and individual practice is highly regimented. You practice everything–batting practice of course, but also fly balls, running, calisthenics, fielding, and individual training with a coach to focus on specific aspects of your own game. You have to get your timing and synchronicity back up to speed as well.

Spring training is analogous to a band getting ready for a tour, spending weeks working on every aspect of the show, from learning new music, to the sound, lighting, staging, order of the tunes, etc. If there's one thing that musicians can learn from ballplayers about spring training, it's this: come prepared. You have an entire team (or band) depending on you. If you show up to spring training out of shape, unfocused, and ill prepared, you bring everybody down. A band or team is only prepared as much as the least prepared member, and there's no worse feeling than starting a season or a tour with doubts and insecurities because the team or the band isn't ready. Finally, remember that it's not only your physical preparedness that's critical–it's your emotional and mental approach at the start of spring training that is vital too. During the off-season, you need to prepare yourself mentally for the start of spring training. Take care of all the personal matters prior to that first dress rehearsal. Be sure you come to that first practice with a clear mind and a positive attitude. It can have an enormous impact on the success of the tour or the season. Great ballplayers and musicians understand this.

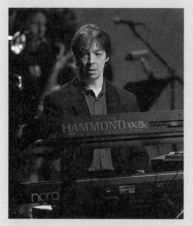

## MINDFUL PRACTICE

by Chris Clark, keyboardist with Bernie Williams, the John Entwistle Band and numerous Broadway musicals, including *Wicked* and *Mamma Mia*

My advice to young performers is: be aware of the quality of your practicing. This will have a big impact on your performance. Pay attention to details, master the materials. Be patient. This is what will bring up your overall skill level as a player, and subsequently as a performer.

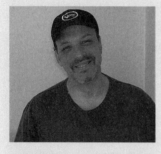

## PROFESSIONALISM

by Loren Harriet, record producer

Over the past twelve years, I have combined the world of sports and music together, and the similarities are remarkable. Having worked with athlete-musicians such as Wayman Tisdale, Bernie Williams, Bronson Arroyo, Dwight Howard, and more, the common theme that I find is the discipline and professional approach that these athlete-musicians take in the recording process. Their level of concentration in the recording studio is incredible.

# 17
# The Competitive Artist

## Understanding healthy competition

*Even as a fierce competitor I try to smile.*
–MAGIC JOHNSON, LOS ANGELES LAKERS

*I love the winning, I can take the losing,*
*but most of all I love to play.*
–BORIS BECKER,
SIX-TIME TENNIS GRAND SLAM SINGLES CHAMPION

*Do you know what my favorite part of the game is?*
*The opportunity to play.*
–MICHAEL SINGLETARY, PRO FOOTBALL HALL OF FAMER

Music was never conceived as competitive sport. However, healthy competition, whether it takes place in a ballpark or in a concert hall, inspires greatness. A competitive spirit is an essential force behind any successful sports franchise–but it plays a vital role in music as well. While baseball has always been a competitive sport, music has its own rich and storied history of competition.

In the 1920s, musical competitions between stride pianists in Harlem were known as "cutting contests." Two of the most famous contestants included James P. Johnson and his rival, Willie "The Lion" Smith. A similar type of cutting contest took place in baseball between pitchers, with one of the most infamous battles occurring in Boston on May 1, 1920, between Leon Cadore of the Brooklyn Robins and Joe Oeschger of the Boston Braves. In what would be unheard of in modern times, the pitchers battled one another for twenty-six innings! In a 1980 interview in *Baseball Research Journal*, Oeschger recounted the game, which almost didn't happen due to rain that day:

> We didn't think the game would be played, but we had to report to the park. It was a Saturday, and I didn't think I would pitch because Manager Stallings usually pitched me on Sundays because I went to church. He always played his hunches. I was happy to get the starting job because Cadore was pitching, and he had beaten me 1–0 in 11 innings earlier in the season. I wanted to even things.

Even things he did! Oeschger and Cadore battled each other to a 1–1 tie in a twenty-six-inning complete game by both pitchers that was dubbed the "Odyssey to Nowhere." Ivy Olson of the Robins begged the umpire to let the game continue just one more inning, seeing the poetry in playing three complete games–twenty-seven innings–in one game, but umpire Barry McCormick made the rare "tie game" call at 6:50 p.m. due to darkness.

In fact, the game took only three hours and fifty minutes (compare this to the nine-inning four-hour-forty-five-minute marathon between the Yankees and the Red Sox that took place on August 18, 2006) and neither pitcher gave up a run in the last twenty innings. Oeschger threw a "mid-game" nine-inning no hitter (with just one walk). Oeschger and Cadore are estimated to have each thrown over 300 pitches. If ever there was a marathon pitchers' duel, Oeschger versus. Cadore was it!

But there would be another duel to emerge seventeen years later in New York, and it didn't occur on the ball field–it took place on the bandstand.

In the 1930s, during the swing era, jazz bands would compete in a "battle of the bands" for supremacy on the stage. The competition was fierce but respectful–even playful (many of the leading bandleaders had their own royal titles–the "King of Swing" (Benny Goodman), the "Duke" (Edward Kennedy Ellington), and the "Count" (William Basie).

The legendary battle of the bands in the swing era reached its peak on Tuesday, May 11, 1937. On this day, the defending world champions, the New York Yankees, took on the Chicago White Sox at Comiskey Park, with Joe DiMaggio and Lou Gehrig in the lineup and Bump Hadley on the mound for the Yankees.

While Gehrig and DiMaggio were taking the field at Comiskey Park to battle the White Sox, another battle was unfolding back in New York, within a mile of Yankee Stadium over at the Savoy Ballroom in Harlem on the corner of 140th Street and Lenox Avenue. The King of Swing, Benny Goodman, and his band were taking the stage in a battle of the bands against drummer Chick Webb and his band. The Savoy had seen nothing like it–a record crowd (some reports estimated it at over 4,000) packed the ballroom to hear these two bands duke it out.

In Chicago, the White Sox pitcher Monty Stratton silenced the Yanks through seven shutout innings. Back in New York, Chick Webb and Benny Goodman battled one another for nearly five hours, the winner to be decided by audience ballot. As the defending champions fell to the White Sox in a 4–1 loss, so too did the "King of Swing" as Chick Webb's band outplayed and outshined Benny Goodman and his legendary band. Goodman's star drummer, Gene Krupa, remarked about Chick Webb, "He just cut me to ribbons. When he really let go, you had a feeling that the entire atmosphere in the place was being charged."

The competition between musicians continued in the late 1970s and early 1980s with a form of competitive recitation, or freestyle rhyming, known as "battle rapping," which originated in the East Coast hip-hop scene. One of the earliest and most famous "battle raps" took place in December 1982 at Harlem World in Manhattan between Kool Moe Dee and Busy Bee Starski. The more sophisticated raps of Kool Moe defeated Busy Bee, and Kool Moe went on to win one of the first Grammys for a rap artist; he was also the first rapper to perform at the Grammys. He made it clear that hip-hop was here to stay and was a force to be reckoned with.

While Kool Moe and Busy Bee were competing in Harlem in 1982, out in the Midwest, the St. Louis Cardinals and the Milwaukee Brewers met for the first time in the World Series. Soon-to-be Hall of Famers Paul Molitor and Robin Yount set two World Series records that year–Molitor with five hits in Game 1 and Yount with two four-hit games. But the MVP went to Cardinals' catcher Darrell Porter, as the Brewers fell to the Cardinals in seven tense games.

So what can we learn from these rivalries and competition among ballplayers and athletes? Well, there's a public fascination about rivalries in baseball (the Red Sox versus the Yankees) and in music (the Beatles versus the Rolling Stones), but too often, the true purpose and nature of a rivalry or competition is lost.

Competition–healthy, positive competition–inspires greatness and instills a sense of accomplishment and gratitude. Red Sox fans taunted by Yankees fans in the Bronx (or vice versa at Fenway) is anathema to the true spirit of competition. Competition, at its purest, instills respect, admiration, and shared joy in having been given the privilege of competing, regardless of who wins or loses. When properly channeled, a competitive spirit bolsters our confidence, tempers our pride, and gives us pause for humility.

Consider this: one of the greatest rivalries that played out on the field occurred on October 3, 1951, in a fierce battle between the New York Giants and the Brooklyn Dodgers for the National League pennant. Bobby Thomson, batting for the Giants, had a 0–1 count with two runners on base in the bottom of the ninth, with the Giants trailing, 2–4. On the mound for the Dodgers was pitcher Ralph Branca, and his next pitch would make history. Thomson drilled a line-drive three-run homer that won the pennant for the Giants–the infamous "Shot heard round the world." Branca was devastated–so too was the entire city of Brooklyn.

But Branca understood the true nature of competition– he and Bobby Thomson went on to become good friends, making frequent television appearances and even performing together, singing a song about the matchup (the song ended with Thomson crooning, "I got the home run," to which Branca chimed in, "yeah, but I got the girl!").

Both Bobby Thomson and Ralph Branca understood the true nature of competition—that with every win comes humility, and with every loss eventually comes the joy at having played one's heart out. Respect, humility, and compassion are all integral to being a great competitor.

## BATTLE OF THE BANDS

by Bernie Williams, Dave Gluck, and Bob Thompson

Without a healthy, competitive, and artistic rivalry, it's quite possible we wouldn't have two of the greatest albums of all time.

Back in the 1960s, the Beatles and the Beach Boys were engaged in an inspired cross-Atlantic artistic rivalry of their own. The Beatles album *Rubber Soul* inspired Brian Wilson to write music for the landmark album *Pet Sounds*—which in turn inspired John Lennon and Paul McCartney to write *Sgt. Pepper*. Even the press-infused rivalry between the Rolling Stones and the Beatles was playful—Mick Jagger and John Lennon were friends—and if you look closely enough at the cover of the Beatles' album *Sgt. Pepper*, there's a Shirley Temple doll sporting a shirt that says, "Welcome the Rolling Stones."

## ARIA

by Manuel Márquez-Sterling, historian

I have two passions in my life: one is baseball and the other is opera. Fortunately enough, they fall in different seasons—opera is in the winter and baseball is in the summer. And people ask me, "How can you like both? They are different." And I say, "Oh no, they are exactly the same thing."

Opera is an epiphanic art, you know; people go to the opera and put up with the recitatives and the tedium waiting for the aria. Now you go to a baseball game and observe what happens: there is no action whatsoever. There is continued tedium. The pitcher has the ball and rubs it, and he's ready to pitch—and the batter steps out—and the pitcher has to wait until he comes back—and then suddenly he hits the ball—and that's the epiphany. Everything comes at that time. It's a moment of great action, and I find the similarity right there.

Besides, the prima donnas that you have in the game are very similar. So, for me, I say when I retire, I would like to get a part-time job in a baseball stadium in the summer and in an opera house in the winter—and that would be heaven for me.

# SEPTEMBER 25, 2001

by Bernie Williams

On September 18, the baseball season resumed after the tragic events of 9/11, and although baseball wasn't foremost on any of our minds, we flew out to Chicago to play the White Sox. As our charter flight took off from LaGuardia Airport, the pilot announced that we were cleared to fly over ground zero at a low altitude—maybe 2,000 feet. We all looked out the windows of the plane in silence. Of all the flights I've taken with the Yankees, the flight to Chicago was one I will never forget.

A week later, we came back to Yankee Stadium—the first game to be played there after 9/11. I could feel the emotional heaviness on the field that night. The Yankees and the Rays were there to win, but even on the field, all of us on both teams realized that this was but a game—and the heroes that night were not ballplayers but the rescue workers from ground zero, who lined up side by side along the baselines with both Rays and Yankees players. It wasn't easy for us that night to experience the joy of the game, but being there with those rescue workers meant the world to us.

The game started an hour late, due to the emotional pregame ceremonies. I managed to crank out two hits, and Jorge Posada and Scott Brosius each had one, but we lost to the fine pitching of Tanyon Sturtze that night, 4–0. In the seventh inning, we learned that Boston had lost to Baltimore, and despite our loss against the Rays, we clinched our fourth straight AL East title. But there was, for the first time in Yankees history, no champagne celebration in the clubhouse that night.

You might wonder how two very competitive teams felt playing that first game at Yankee Stadium after the tragedy. Scott Brosius said before the game, "I think this is one step to getting things back to normal. It will take a long time to heal the wounds. Maybe this can be part of that." Tanyon Sturtze of the Rays said it best: "Everyone was just playing for New York. We were playing for New York—and the Yankees were playing for New York."

## OUT BUT NOT DOWN

by Bernie Williams

The record stood for fifty-seven years—not since Johnny Broaca on June 25, 1934, had a New York Yankee ever struck out five times in one game. Fast-forward fifty-seven years.

I made my major league debut with the Yankees on July 7, 1991—and it only took me forty-five days in the majors to break that record. I was fanned four times by Bret Saberhagen (and once by "Storm" Davis) of the Kansas City Royals. I gotta tip my hat to Bret and Storm.

To put it in perspective, if you're a major league ballplayer, you have to really be abysmal to strike out five times in one game. It's actually a very difficult thing to do, but somehow—I managed to pull it off.

So imagine what I was thinking after that game? Did I feel lousy?

Well, it's hard not to feel that way when you break a record that nobody ever wants to break.

But was I thinking, "Am I going to be sent down to the minors?" and "Is my career in baseball over?" Not a chance!

If there was one feeling I experienced above everything else, it was this: fierce resolve and utter determination. After that game, all I could think was, "Give me one more chance!" When I got to the stadium the next day, all I wanted to see was my name in the lineup, because if it was, I knew I would turn things around. And I did. I went two for four against the Blue Jays.

# 18
# The Success of Failing

## Why your approach to failure is key to your success

*People succeed when they realize that their failures are the preparation for their victories.*

–RALPH WALDO EMERSON

It's odd that the word *failure*–for musicians and athletes–has such negative connotations. The root of the word, from the French word *faillir* simply means an omission of occurrence–an outcome that was not expected. But most of us in sports and the arts use a more common definition: lack of success. Nothing could be further from the truth. There is success in failure, and there is even failure in success. Sometimes both happen simultaneously–your team can still win the World Series even though you batted .100 and were in a slump.

Baseball is a game of failure. There exists no other competitive sport where an individual is doomed to failure at such a high percentage (an average ballplayer batting .250 will fail every three out of four at bats). Professional musicians, however, perform at a much lower rate of failure by necessity. A classical musician performing with a major symphony orchestra, such as the New York Philharmonic, might have a "batting average" of .950–unheard of in baseball. Yet the commonality we witness among both younger musicians and ballplayers is their approach to failure.

How often have you seen a dejected young musician or athlete walk off the field or stage, head hanging low, after not hitting the ball, not successfully playing that difficult passage on their instrument, or just not performing well and failing to rise to the occasion? While it's a perfectly normal reaction to feel disappointed, especially after striking out or missing a note, feelings of failure should not be part of your mental and emotional vocabulary. Ever.

So, what should be your frame of mind after you struck out on that fastball high and inside? What should be your thinking as you leave the stage, head down, feeling dejected?

As a ballplayer, you have to realize that no matter how good you are, you are going to fail a considerable amount of the time and you have to be able to learn from it, put it behind you, and use what you gained from the experience to improve. Musicians need to understand this too.

There is nothing negative about it—failure is a moment of unique opportunity that instructs, informs, and makes it possible for us to improve, so long as we understand it as such. It is the very act of failing that is at the basis of every great athlete and musician. That's why we like the less common definition of the word: an outcome that was not expected. When something unexpected occurs, it is an opportunity for us to become familiar with it, learn from it, and let it inform our practice and increase our consistency and skill. Few young ballplayers and musicians grasp this—that failure is actually a prerequisite for improvement and success, and is the mark of every true champion.

The Rock and Roll Hall of Fame and the National Baseball Hall of Fame pay tribute to the greatest players ever. Each musician and ballplayer had a unique, singular experience that brought them to that moment of excellence, of surpassing the bar, and being a member of baseball's and music's most elite clubs. Yet the one common denominator among every member of the Hall of Fame (rock or baseball) is that each person, at some point in their lives, experienced failure. No one is exempt. Even the great Babe Ruth went through hitting slumps—and not every Beatles song was a number-one hit (although any baseball player would love to have the Beatles' batting average when it came to writing number-one hit songs).

# THE SUCCESS OF FAILING

There are many paths to excellence and greatness, but all these paths pass through failure at some point. It is precisely at this moment, when any rational person would feel discouraged, that the greatest players paradoxically feel encouraged.

One of the most inspiring examples of handling failure positively began back in 2001, during the final game of the World Series against the Arizona Diamondbacks. The great Yankees closer Mariano Rivera, who holds the major league postseason records for saves and earned run average, blew a save in the bottom of the ninth inning by allowing Luis Gonzalez's bloop single with the bases loaded to score the winning run. Granted, we could all put baseball in perspective that year–the tragic events of 9/11 had occurred just eight weeks earlier–but the loss was nonetheless heartbreaking for the Yankees, for Yankees fans, and most of all for Mo.

All of us have experienced failure, but imagine how it must have felt for Mariano Rivera to have the World Series championship slip through his fingers? For many, it would have been beyond discouraging–it'd be devastating and perhaps career altering. A younger pitcher, with less experience and a different attitude, might have never recovered from the loss.

During this time, was Mo disappointed? Absolutely. Did he get discouraged?

Sure, but the next day he was beyond the disappointment, focusing instead on how he could use what happened to his advantage–to learn from it, to improve and continue to dominate the game.

But the World Series loss was only the beginning of what would turn out to be a difficult 2002 season for Mo–he was on the disabled list three times, and pitched only forty-six innings. He also missed the first month of the 2003 season as well. There was talk of Mo having lost his dominance. Did any of these setbacks cause Mo to become discouraged? Not a chance!

When Mariano Rivera returned a month into the 2003 season, he was as dominant as ever, recording forty saves in forty-six opportunities with a 1.66 ERA in sixty-four games in the 2003 regular season. But that was just the beginning.

In what would be one of the Yankees' defining games, Mo delivered what many believe to be one of the greatest postseason performances ever, during Game 7 of the 2003 American League Championship Series against the Boston Red Sox. With the score tied, 5–5, in the ninth inning, Joe Torre summoned Mo. As the door to center field opened and Mo entered to the soundtrack of Metallica's "Enter Sandman," the ovation was thunderous.

What was about to unfold would be one of the most tense, on-the-edge-of-your-seat experiences in baseball history. Brilliantly pitching three scoreless innings, Mo kept the Red Sox in check, setting the stage for Aaron Boone to hit an eleventh-inning walk-off home run (coincidentally, less than a mile from where Bobby Thompson hit his Game 7 "Shot Heard Round the World") and the Yankees won the pennant. It was an amazing performance, preceded by a difficult 2002 season, coupled with the loss in the World Series in 2001. Mo had triumphed again, and while the Yankees eventually lost the 2003 World Series to the Florida Marlins, Mo allowed only one earned run in sixteen innings pitched that postseason.

So what does Mariano Rivera have in common with every young ballplayer or musician trying to excel and be the best? Failure. But Mo has something else: a deep understanding that failure is nothing but an opportunity dressed in a poor disguise called disappointment and setback. The next time you walk off the stage or field not having excelled–you struck out, got nervous and gave a less-than-stellar performance, or simply didn't perform well–don't ever let negative thoughts and discouragement take hold. Step back from the experience, learn from it, take solace in all of those professional musicians and ballplayers who have walked in the very same shoes you are now walking in, and be encouraged.

Failure, in the minds of great players, is a very powerful and positive force that can be the start of something great. The Chinese philosopher Confucius said it best: "Our greatest glory is not in never falling, but in rising every time we fall." Mariano Rivera lives this philosophy every day.

## UNDERSTANDING FEAR

by Don Greene

Fear is an emotional defense against loss. Athletes and performing artists share three main fears: injuries, mistakes, and failure. They also fear ego loss (embarrassment).

Most people are taught to live in fear and reinforce it on their own. Fear is the energy that contracts, closes down, runs, hides, hoards, and harms. Fear inhibits, restricts, delays, or prevents movement in a positive direction.

Everybody has fear when approaching something new or challenging. Yet so many are doing things despite the fear, so fear must not be the problem. The real issue is what we do or don't do in response to the fear. The "big fear" is that you won't be able to handle it, whatever it is.

Some people respond to fear from a position of powerlessness, paralysis, and resignation. They don't move at all or fall back in a negative direction. The secret of handling fear is to move from a position of powerlessness and paralysis to a position of power, courage, and action.

Face the fear. Take action and move in a positive direction past the fear. Practice doing the things you fear in small, progressive steps. After a while, the fear will become irrelevant.

If you're a musician or competitive athlete, the fear will never go away as long as you continue to grow. You stretch your capabilities and expand your comfort zone by taking calculated risks. The only way to feel better is to go out and do what you fear.

You are going to experience fear when in unfamiliar territory or when taking risks. But pushing through the fear is less frightening than living with the bigger underlying fear that comes from the feeling of powerlessness.

Here are some key points to remember about fear:

- What you fear you attract into your reality.
- That which you fear strongly you will experience.
- Confront the fear and it begins to disappear.
- Bravery is not the absence of fear, but doing what you fear.
- Do the thing you fear in progressive steps.
- Take calculated risks at the right time.

- Building courage is like strengthening a muscle.
- Courage comes from repetition and by taking increased risks.
- Commit to go for it ahead of time.
- Act as if you have all the courage in the world.
- Keep your sense of humor.
- If you can laugh at your fears, they diminish significantly.

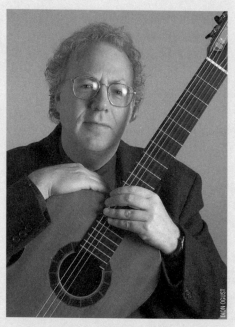

## ADVICE FROM THE BENCH

by Frederic Hand, Grammy-nominated guitarist and composer, guitarist with the Metropolitan Opera

I had a teacher in college who said to me once, "When you get a bad review—just forget about it. And when you get a good review—forget about that too." What he meant was not to get too high or too low about yourself—just concentrate on what you're doing. Work hard and the results will take care of themselves.

When it comes to concentration and focus, remember this—each time we allow our minds to disengage and drift off, we're allowing a muscle to go weak. We can strengthen our ability to focus by returning our attention back to the activity, over and over again. It truly is like building up a muscle—an internalized, focusing muscle that strengthens our concentration as we use it.

Practice does not necessarily make perfect. It does, however, make whatever you practice permanent.

When you see ballplayers excelling, they are having fun. I remind my students to enjoy the experience when they play. We've been given a wonderful gift and it is a great privilege to spend our lives doing what we love.

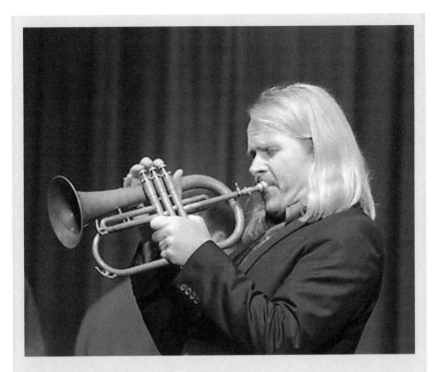

## BATTING .000

by Bob Thompson

Early on in my career as a musician, I used to get incredibly nervous before performing. I excelled in the practice room, but failed miserably in front of an audience. While in high school, I played a solo with the school band, and I was so nervous that my trumpet acquired this terribly unnatural vibrato–the performance was a disaster. At home, I could play that solo from memory, but put me in front of a crowd and I froze. I would have made a great poster child for performance anxiety.

When I arrived at the Eastman School of Music in Rochester, New York, to further my musical studies, my trumpet teacher had all the new students get up and perform a solo in front of all the other students on the first day of class. I was terrified. When I got up to play, it was a repeat of that disastrous high school performance. I left class that day, went back to my dorm room, and remember looking at myself in the mirror and saying, "You shouldn't be here–you just don't have what it takes." As much as I loved music–which I excelled at in the practice room–I started to think about changing my major. Perhaps I'd be better off studying English, history, or business. Suddenly the phone rang. It was my teacher.

She said, "Look–you're going to graduate from here and you're going to be a great performer, even if I have to put you through hell and make you get in front of an audience every day during your time here."

And she almost did just that. Every week, I'd be forced to get up and play in front of the class. It became my worst nightmare and I failed miserably each time. But after two months of "bombing" in class every Wednesday, something profoundly strange happened. I started to laugh at my nervousness.

I'd think, "Oh, it's Wednesday–time for my weekly public performance disaster." When I played poorly in front of the other students, I'd laugh it off. I honestly didn't care about being nervous anymore. It was at this moment that I simply stopped taking myself so seriously. I became the Bob Uecker of trumpet players–I'd get up in front of the other students and say, "You all know the piece I'm about to play, but I'm going to tell you the title of it anyway in case you don't recognize it." I could have written a thesis on "proactive apathy."

After the first semester, something even stranger occurred–I started to look forward to those Wednesday performances. I actually enjoyed and embraced performing in front of people. I started to give recitals, came out of my shell, and took every chance I could to perform in front of people. Within a year, performing in front of people became a joy–and slowly but surely, I began to excel at it.

My concentration and focus improved, and I started to think and perform more creatively. That one year had radically altered my approach to practicing, and I finally understood that performing involves an entirely different mindset than practicing. I was emboldened–if someone had come along and said, "Dude, Carnegie Hall–tomorrow night!" I would have answered, "Bring it on. I'm ready!" To this day, it was the most profound change that's occurred in my professional life.

Since that time, I've toured around the globe and performed hundreds of concerts, and–get this–the thing I had feared the most became the thing I loved doing the most. A few years back, I stood onstage at the Ravinia Festival in Chicago, about to conduct an open-air concert with the Chicago Symphony Orchestra. I turned around to talk to the audience, and there were 6,000 people spread out on the grass–yet I was relaxed, focused, and most importantly–enjoying the moment.

# THE SUCCESS OF FAILING

We are all given certain gifts—some people are born with resilience under pressure and others have to work hard to acquire it. My advice to young ballplayers and musicians who struggle with performance anxiety is this: run towards what you fear, because it will make you stronger. If you get nervous in front of people and in pressure situations, give yourself more opportunities to be nervous. After a while, you'll embrace the nervousness—and learn to positively channel it into a great performance. I still get nervous—but now it's like an old friend who comes backstage to the dressing room before the show to wish me well and ensure I'm amped up.

Finally, understand that you can't get to this level—unless you're naturally born with it (which I clearly wasn't)—without spending considerable time performing. Repetition is key—a ballplayer in high school might play upwards of forty games a season, whereas young musicians rarely have this frequency of performance opportunities. Performing in front of people is truly an acquired skill that you can only learn through doing it—continuously.

# 19
# Band on the Run

How great teams and bands develop
positive team spirit

*It is amazing what can be accomplished when
it doesn't matter who gets the credit.*
–HARRY S. TRUMAN

*The secret is to work less as individuals and more as a
team.*
*As a coach, I play not my eleven best, but my best eleven.*
–KNUTE ROCKNE

*You're looking for players whose name on the front of
the sweater is more important than the one on the back.
I look for these players to play hard, to play smart, and
to represent their country.*
–HERB BROOKS,
COACH OF 1980 U.S. OLYMPIC HOCKEY TEAM

It was 1996 and we were the unknown underdogs. At the
time, the Yankees were a team of blue-collar players with
no superstars–in hindsight, we embodied the definition of
the word *team*. We fully trusted and believed in each other's
ability, and were quick to prop up a teammate when needed. We trusted each other, our staff, and especially our new
manager, Joe Torre. We played our game and game strategy
the way Joe Torre told us to. We stuck to his plan–we played
a lot of "small ball" and although we were not superstars, we
were collectively a balanced and fundamentally sound team.

There was nothing special about us on paper or in the
stats that would leap off the page at you. We simply worked

hard and kept our heads down as we gained physical and mental resilience by grinding it out each day. And we never gave up—ever. We'd go into the ninth inning of a game, down by three runs with two outs, and there was no one on our team—not a soul—who didn't believe we would come back and find a way to win.

It's been said that winning is the great equalizer—and when your boss was Mr. Steinbrenner—*The Boss*—winning was job number one. However, the true measure of our team back in those days wasn't in the winning—the winning was simply the effect. The true measure was how we reacted when we lost and how we handled adversity. Teams—like individual players—go through collective slumps and this is when individual teammates show their true colors. When we were in a slump, we never played with desperation, nor did anyone play selfishly. We came together, hunkered down, and focused. We concentrated solely on our approach, not the results.

For instance, if we had a guy on second with no outs, it didn't matter who was batting: all of us knew that our primary responsibility was not to do too much to prove our worth as individuals, but to simply move the runner over by hitting the ball to the right side. It sounds simple, but in reality, it's very difficult unless you're truly a team.

We also started to feel like a team—and we started to feed off each other's successes. It's like playing with jazz musicians—if somebody is having a great night and they're soloing—and the crowd is going nuts—a great band will feed off of that and support the soloist. It's no longer about one person—it's about the music—and when the soloist builds and builds their solo, and then there's this moment where everybody is like, "Yeah!"—it makes everybody feel great. That's what it felt like with the Yankees starting in 1996—if a ball was hit to right field and Paul O'Neil fired it to Tino Martinez ,who fired it home to Posada to tag the runner, we'd all feel like, "Yeah! Here we come!" We were an emphatic team—and we truly rejoiced in one another's successes.

When we were down as a team, we simply focused and

reduced our game to accomplishing only the task at hand. It was a "less is more" strategy, the exact opposite of what your intellect would tell you to do. We became like Zen masters of baseball—we were selfless, and this made us all the more stronger. And we supported one another.

One of the characteristics I've noticed among great ballplayers is their ability to inspire those around them to perform at their utmost potential. They become a force in the clubhouse, and their energy is contagious—they bring about the best in you and your teammates. They're genuinely concerned for your mental, physical, and spiritual well-being. They want the best for you, and they demonstrate that through their actions on the field and their demeanor and presence in the clubhouse.

Don Mattingly, the captain of the Yankees at the time, was like this. I remember him saying to me once in my first few years in the majors, "Bernie, I don't care what you do off the field, but when you come here—play with everything you have." He became a role model for me in my early years. There's no greater feeling than coming to work each day and being part of a team that believes in each other and will do anything to prop up those who are struggling and having a bad day.

The manifestation of this team, its philosophy, and approach came to fruition in 1998. We were no longer unknown and there was an aura about us—an intimidation factor—because other teams saw how locked in and focused we were and how we acted as a team, especially when we were down. We won a franchise record-breaking 114 regular season games, finishing twenty-two games in front of the second-place Red Sox. After the postseason in which we won the World Series, we had won an unprecedented 125 games.

There were no weak links in the Yankees that year, yet we weren't superstars. Consider this—Scott Brosius joined the Yankees that year—and the prior year he batted .203 for Oakland. By the close of the 1998 season, Brosius batted .300 during the season and won the World Series MVP. We didn't have the superstars of the 1927 "Murder's Row" Yankees—Combs, Koenig, Meusel, Lazzeri, Gehrig, and Ruth—but we played the game as a team.

I have taken this amazing experience of the Yankees playing as a team during this period and brought it to the stage. We're not a band of superstars—we rehearse and work together as a team. The history of music is littered with great bands that broke up because of egos, disagreements, selfishness, and a lack of respect for the other players. It's important to put the game and the music above yourself in order to make great art. The collaborative process—of truly working together for the greater good of the music—is a skill set that every musician needs to learn if they're going to succeed. Great art happens when we let go of ourselves and work together.

## IT TAKES A BAND—IT TAKES A TEAM

by Mario Cuomo, former governor of New York, reprinted by permission from *Baseball*, a film by Ken Burns

The idea of community, the idea of coming together, we're still not good at that in this country. We talk about it a lot. In moments of crisis, we're magnificent at it—the Depression and Franklin D. Roosevelt lifting himself from his wheelchair to lift this nation from its knees—at those moments, we understand community and helping one another.

In baseball you do that all the time—you can't win it alone. You can be the best pitcher in baseball, but somebody has to get you a run to win the game. It is a community activity—you need all nine players helping one another.

I love bunt plays—I love the idea of the bunt—the sacrifice bunt. Even the word *sacrifice* is good—giving yourself up for the good of the whole. That's Jeremiah—that's thousands of years of wisdom. You find your own good in the good of the whole—and your own individual fulfillment is found in the success of the community—the Bible tried to do that and didn't teach you. Baseball did.

# WINNING ON THE ROAD

........................................................................................................

by Bernie Williams, Dave Gluck, and Bob Thompson

........................................................................................................

Being on tour with a ball club or a band can be challenging. Beyond the variables of playing in different stadiums and arenas, the constant travel can be grueling and–if you're not careful and don't prepare yourself properly–can lead to a host of problems. You may have come off a great home stand, but now you're on the road, playing in other teams' backyards. You don't have the comforts of home, you're in unfamiliar places, and you're away from your loved ones and family. While there's initial excitement about traveling to new places, the reality is that you're on a business trip, not a vacation–and you need to take care of business.

Being on the road with a band or a ball club brings a total change of environment to your "at home" routine–including the ballpark, the climate, hotels, buses, restaurants, etc. For instance, if you're in a playoff game verses the Colorado Rockies and you're not prepared, your stamina is going to be affected due to the high altitude. The high altitude makes fly balls travel about 10 percent farther, there's a slight reduction in the ability of pitchers to throw effective breaking balls, and baseballs dry out quicker (they have to be kept in humidors, much like cigars).

The result is that you're faced with a number of new variables that you don't have at home. It's part of the reason why there's a home-field advantage to begin with–the home team is acclimated to the variables, whereas the away team may not be. The same is true for touring musicians–playing in unfamiliar venues where there's a different stage, equipment, sound system, lighting, etc. can wreak havoc with touring musicians if they're not prepared.

Life on the road is a time to be focused and prepared. If you want to perform at your best, it's not a time to be partying all night. In fact, the opposite is true–you need to work harder, stay in your routine, eat well, and take care of yourself. There's nothing worse than getting sick or injured while on the road. You're also traveling in close quarters with your band mates or teammates–so be respectful of one another. Above all, enjoy the experience–there's nothing quite like touring with a band or a ball club.

# 20
# Leader of the Band

## The nature of leadership

No band or team can be successful without leadership, whether it's the band manager, the team manager, or someone within the band or team. I know that a good part of my success as a ballplayer was a result of good leadership–I had someone whom I could follow and look up to and who believed in me. Joe Torre's best quality as a manager was his people skills–he knew that each player on the team was different and he took the time to understand the personalities of players–that was his greatest gift. He wasn't a cookie-cutter manager and his approach wasn't generic.

For instance, Joe would leave me alone–he knew I would take care of business and do what I needed to do because that was part of my makeup. He also knew when it was best for the team for a player to focus on himself and when it was better for him to focus on the team–like bunts, for example. Joe never wanted me to bunt–his approach to me was that I should focus on what I did best. I once tried to bunt in a game to get a runner on, and Joe came up to me afterwards and said, "Bernie, if I catch you trying to bunt one more time, I'll fine you! You serve the team better by being Bernie!"

With other players, Joe took a different approach. He had a level of sensitivity that enabled him to bring out the best in every personality on the team. That was his most talented trait. He also had a team-based philosophy–the Yankees were a team of great players who wanted to play all the time and there was a level of talent and nuance to how he managed everyone's playing time. Joe was successful in convincing players to buy into the team philosophy, that the team came first and the players second. It sounds simple, but the level of skill needed to pull this off successfully—without alienating anyone—is remarkable.

A great manager is a mental athlete—managing the game and the players, understanding what makes everyone tick and what will make each player improve. A great manager is part leader and part psychologist and knows that, regardless of what physical state you are in, you're not going to perform to your potential if you're not mentally confident. Inspiring mental confidence is critical—especially when it comes to risk taking. It's here that a manager comes into play—if your disposition as a human being is to naturally be cautious or reserved, a manager can have a huge impact on your psyche when it comes to taking chances on the field. If your manager believes in you—believes you can steal second—then you'll be that much more confident when you're leading off the bag on first.

Great managers also inspire humility in their players—he or she sets the tone for the entire team in this way. But managers also understand the difference between humility and weakness. A player that appears overly humble in the midst of a slump might need to be coached to turn it up a notch. Above all, great managers inspire players to continue learning new things and to be open to new ideas. There are players who have arrived at a certain plateau—maybe they came off a great season and the manager senses they're getting a bit too overconfident. A good manager might take the player aside and remind them not to get complacent, lest they find themselves falling into a slump.

Leadership is just as important in music, perhaps more so. A great conductor, like Gustavo Dudamel, who leads the Los Angeles Philharmonic, is an inspired leader. The great Count Basie and the legendary Duke Ellington were natural leaders too. Every up-and-coming rock band needs leadership, from within the band and from without.

The Beatles had an inspired leader in their manager, Brian Epstein, who was instrumental in the rise in popularity of the Fab Four. He was there at the very beginning of the Beatles when they first formed in Liverpool, saw their potential, and never waivered in his faith and commitment to them.

He knew his role and never interfered artistically with the band—limiting his work to building the image and reputation and doggedly pursuing the band's first record contract. He was revered—was generous and kind—and acted as the patriarch of the Beatles family.

A good manager has a great rapport, a sense of camaraderie, and even a bit of humor when it's appropriate. There was one time where I had to go to the team doctor—I had a tooth that was really bothering me. I was in Joe Torre's office, waiting for the doctor, and Joe said, "Bernie, I'm leaving now, so why don't you wait and lay down on my couch until the doctor arrives."

So I did and Joe got up to leave. He opened the door, and then he paused for a moment, turned around, and said, "But, Bernie, don't stay too long on that couch—the team might think you're my favorite."

I looked up and said, "But, Joe, they already know I am!"

It was a minor exchange of words between us—a bit of jesting between manager and player—but it is those small moments that you treasure and that inspire you to do your manager proud when you're on the field.

I was asked once, "Whom would you rather have as tour manager for your band—Joe Torre or Don Zimmer?" I replied, "Definitely Joe, but I'd want Zim there as stage manager, letting people backstage and kicking people out. He'd be good at that."

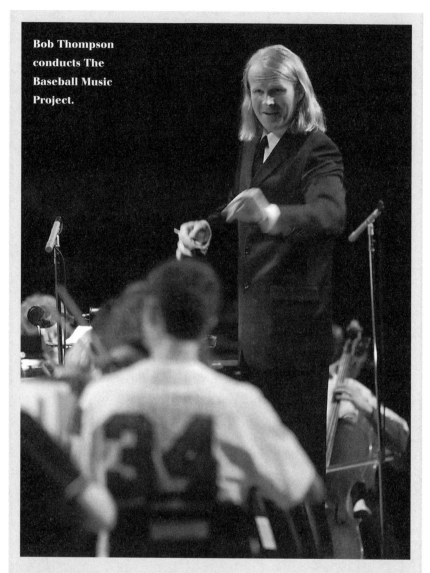

Bob Thompson conducts The Baseball Music Project.

# A PODIUM AND A PLATE

by Bob Thompson

I've had the privilege over the years of conducting some of America's great orchestras in presenting The Baseball Music Project with Hall of Famer Dave Winfield—including the Detroit, Phoenix, Seattle, and Houston Symphony Orchestras, among others. Great orchestras function like great baseball teams. Getting into a major orchestra is as competitive as making it to the majors–an opening in a major orchestra will result in perhaps hundreds of applicants who audition, going through a series of "tryouts" until a victor emerges. These top musicians have spent thousands of hours honing their craft. Each is a unique, talented artist with his or her own personality and style. No two violinists are alike, just as no two ballplayers are the same.

The role of the conductor in an orchestra is not unlike the manager of a baseball team. You have a team of great players, and you want to inspire and bring the best out in all of them. In most cases, I'll have but two rehearsals to put an entire concert together, so when I show up, I need to be prepared and concise and have a game plan. Most importantly, I need to manage the rehearsals and be efficient as possible. If I do these things well, I'll earn the respect of the musicians–and if I, in turn, show respect to them, we end up making great music and having fun too.

One of the highlights for me was conducting the Milwaukee Symphony in the summer of 2010 in a ceremony at Miller Park, honoring players such as Hank Aaron, Robin Yount, Frank Robinson, and Jackie Robinson. I was conducting music from *The Natural* and *Field of Dreams* as Rachel Robinson and all these great players stood onstage with the orchestra–it was a humbling experience and a moment I'll cherish for many years.

In one of the more lighthearted moments, I was conducting the Detroit Symphony, and during a break in the rehearsal, Dave Winfield went to the podium, picked up my baton, and started waving it–imagining he was me. I said, "Dave, how about I teach you to conduct and you can teach me to hit?" I ended up giving him a mini-conducting lesson on the spot, and that night at the concert, he became the first Hall of Famer to ever conduct a major orchestra, debuting with the encore, "Take Me Out to the Ball Game." He did so well that he got a standing ovation.

# 21
# Moving Forward

## How to embrace change

*You count on it, rely on it to buffer the passage of time, to keep the memory of sunshine and high skies alive, and then just when the days are all twilight, when you need it most, it stops. Today . . . it stopped, and summer was gone.*
–BART GIAMATTI, "THE GREEN FIELDS OF THE MIND"

*I knew when my career was over. In 1965 my baseball card came out with no picture.*
–BOB UECKER

*You can play music forever.*
*It's not like playing baseball.*
–MICK JAGGER

*A life is not important except in the impact it has on other lives.*
–JACKIE ROBINSON

In my last few years as a Yankee, I'd do something special at the end of every season: I'd wait until everyone had left and picked up their things and then I'd head to the clubhouse to my locker and pick my things up, after which I'd walk out onto the field of Yankee Stadium to be alone. It's a rare feeling to be on the field of Yankee Stadium all by yourself with no one in the stands. I'd walk around in the infield, then head out to the patch of grass that was my home for sixteen years. I'd look in on home plate, and I'd imagine the crowd– there I am in the on-deck circle. There I am at the plate. I imagined I'm hitting one more home run.

The old Yankee Stadium was my friend and partner–it was alive and animate. So after every season during my last five, six years, I'd spend time alone with it for a few minutes. Then I'd say good-bye, walk off the field, and head out into the parking lot, and drive home to be with my family. The last time I did this was in October 2006–but I didn't know leaving the stadium that day that I would never again return to the field in pinstripes.

Musicians and baseball players share this in common: their lives are often filled with transitions. It's rare for a major league ballplayer to spend his entire career playing for the same team, and it's rare for a musician to spend their entire career with just one band. Those players and musicians that have been privileged–as I was with the Yankees for sixteen years–to spend an entire career with just one organization are few and far between. The Rolling Stones are still together–as are U2 and Aerosmith. But many bands–like Led Zeppelin, the Police, and the Beatles–parted company–although both the Police and Zeppelin reunited within the past few years, and that's always a great thing to see.

Ballplayers and musicians switch teams and bands, and some move on to other aspects of the game or business. Quincy Jones was a marvelous musician but had an even more successful career as an arranger and producer. Many retired ballplayers stay in baseball–as managers and coaches or working in the front office. But it's not quite the same–everyone dreams of turning back the clock to the summer of our youth–we wish ballplayers were like musicians, and we could continue performing like Mick Jagger or Paul Mc-Cartney well into our sixties and beyond. Baseball is unlike music in this respect–careers last but for the summer of our lives, and then we're left to face autumn alone, without the team. A recent study found that the average career of a major league ballplayer is only 5.6 years.

Outside of baseball, the days of starting a job out of college and continuing on with the same organization, like many of our fathers did, is rare. The average person will have seven to ten jobs in their lifetime. Many of us face career transitions, but those in baseball are perhaps the hardest. Unlike musicians, we can't continue to perform like we did—and while I'm sure playing at an old timer's game can be a lot of fun, it's simply not the same.

I've been extremely blessed in transitioning out of baseball—in part because of my supportive family, but also because music has always been a big part of my life—and now I get to do it full-time.

But there is something else that was even more critical in transitioning—I grew up understanding that a career should never define who you are. Relationships define who you are. No matter what you choose to do, there is one thing I can promise: you are going to be in a position to make a positive impact on somebody's life. And there is nothing more important than that.

So remember this: if you define yourself by who you are, and not what you do, then you can change what you do and you'll still be who you are.

I've had the opportunity to be around a number of great musicians and ballplayers that made it to "the top" of their profession. They all share a rare and rather strange byproduct of their success on the field or on the stage: fame and fortune. They end up becoming celebrities, known by thousands, if not millions. They have adoring fans and get VIP treatment wherever they go. It can all go to your head if you're not careful.

Every young musician or ballplayer dreams of making it big, yet few ever get the opportunity. But is this what is really important in the short time we are on this planet? Is success really about fame, fortune, and being the best? Or is there something larger, more important? Is the game or the music entirely about you and what people think of you?

In other words, with the God-given talent you've been blessed with, are you using it as a means or an ends? Is it all simply about World Series rings, Grammy Awards, and the notoriety that goes with them? If you didn't have music or baseball, what would be important to you? An MVP (Most

Valuable Player) is not always the same thing as an MVP (Most Valuable Person).

We've all seen how fame and success–the two things every young ballplayer and musician dreams about–work both ways. There are those who are humbled by it and acknowledge it for what it is–something temporal and to be used to raise the human condition. And then there are those who get consumed by their own success–engaging in excess, losing track of who they are (or perhaps they never really knew), and ending up with lives that have been sidetracked.

Unfortunately, there's a darker side to baseball and music, where tragically a number of talented young musicians and ballplayers end up with careers derailed because of addiction, depression, or personal or financial pressures. The list of rock musicians whose lives ended tragically and prematurely is filled with names like Jim Morrison, Kurt Cobain, Jimi Hendrix, Janis Joplin, and Keith Moon. There are a number of former major league players who are no longer with us either because of these factors.

The desire to be the best–to be great–should never be an end goal in your career–it should be the means to a higher end. Using your talents should ultimately bring joy to your life–but more importantly–to those around you. If that isn't happening, then you need to take stock of who you are and what is keeping you from truly experiencing the joy of success. Musicians and ballplayers share a unique bond that is at the heart of what makes both professions so very special: nearly every great musician and ballplayer started at a very young age, and it wasn't for the fame or glory, but for the love of music and a love of the game.

There is a comical line from the film *Fever Pitch* where the actor Jimmy Fallon (who plays a die-hard Boston Red Sox fan in the movie) is asked, "You love the Red Sox, but have they ever loved you back?" Therein lies a deeper question: Do you as a musician or ballplayer truly acknowledge and appreciate those people that have come out to see you play? Is it a nuisance to deal with fans or do you understand that, at the end of the day, there's no difference between you and another human being, no matter what success, fame, or fortune has been bestowed upon you? Without those fans taking time out of their lives to see you perform and share in your gift, it would be a very empty performance indeed.

Understanding your core purpose–your *raison d'être*–for being on this planet, along with a deep understanding of your core values as a human being, is vital to your success on the field or on the stage. The greatest players–those that we hold up as heroes–like Ruth, DiMaggio, and Gehrig–were all good, decent people who had a healthy sense of self, even in the face of adversity. Babe Ruth could laugh at himself. Joe DiMaggio was pure elegance who understood the power of silence. And then there was Lou Gehrig, a humble and courageous man, who stood before a packed Yankee Stadium at the age of thirty-six with the knowledge that he didn't have long to live, and said with the utmost sincerity, "Today I consider myself the luckiest man on the face of the earth."

It is imperative that young musicians and ballplayers study the lives of great players like Jackie Robinson and Lou Gehrig and look at what they did to impact the lives of others, not just what they did on the field. There is no doubt that, had these legends never played the game, they would have been heroes in some other profession, and certainly in their personal lives.

Ask yourself, "By what criteria do I measure my self-esteem?" Is a player that never got past AA ball any less than a Hall of Famer? Is a music teacher at an elementary school any less than a rock star?

Consider this: back in 1976, an amateur musician and itinerant music teacher named Hans Fenger started a school music program in Langley, a small town in western Canada. Armed with just a microphone, a tape recorder, and a school gymnasium as a recording studio, he made 200 copies of a vinyl record of his students singing songs by the Beach Boys, Paul McCartney, David Bowie, and others–to give to parents, teachers, and friends. The album lay dormant until a record producer discovered it in an old vinyl record shop and released it commercially in 2001–and this long-lost school project ended up on many a Top-10 list, was lauded by David Bowie, and prompted a VH1 special reuniting those students after twenty-five years. Or consider Gregg Breinberg, a music teacher at PS 22 in Staten Island, New York, who has been directing an elementary school chorus for the past decade. He started posting video clips on YouTube, and to date, their videos have been watched over 30 million times, which led to the chorus performing at the White House and at the Academy Awards. Gregg Breinberg and Hans Fenger may not have achieved rock star status, but in the hearts of all those students they touched through music, they are, indeed, rock stars.

How do you react to failure? Even when your personal life is pleasant and stable, the game of baseball is designed to make you fail seven out of ten times (and that's if you're good at it). How do you handle criticism? Professional musicians and athletes alike are constantly tempted to read critiques and commentaries of their performance on the stage or on the field. Reviews can inflate your ego one day and send you into a depression the next—but only if your entire sense of self-esteem is tied to what others think of you.

Ultimately, you want to have a solid sense of self so that you're able to accept the praise and the criticism, along with the wisdom to temper both. You have no real control over anything that happens in your life or what people think of you—you can only control your preparation and your attitude.

Great players will be the same people regardless of the outcome of their performance. They don't change. They are passionate, but they remain even-keeled. The negative aspects of their lives wash off of them like rain off the backs of ducks. Derek Jeter is a great example of this—he looks adversity right in the eye and chuckles at it. He's consistently unflappable—and his attitude is contagious.

Keep a positive attitude and have fun doing what you do. Don't be afraid to take risks—if you don't take enough of them, you'll miss out on a lot of great moments life has to offer you. Get used to stumbling a bit—you'll gain your footing and learn from it.

# MOVING FORWARD

With every home run comes joy—and with every great song comes a moment of bliss. Above all, make the most of your journey.

# 22
# Little League

Encouraging children in sports and music

*My fondest memories of the game are as a kid playing catch with my brother, testing our arms for accuracy. My brother and I still play catch today, just like we did then. Baseball keeps us young.*
—DAVE WINFIELD,
HALL OF FAMER AND FORMER NEW YORK YANKEE; HOST
AND NARRATOR FOR THE BASEBALL MUSIC PROJECT

As a child growing up in Puerto Rico, I had very supportive parents. They were demanding but nurturing—they pushed my brother (who is a classical cellist) and me hard and expected results from us. They devoted a lot of time to us—they were there at all the events, games, track meets, concerts, and school projects. Not only were they physically present, but they were also fully engaged and involved in our lives. Even though they both had full-time careers (my mom was a principal and my dad was a merchant marine), they were there for us—they had a well-thought-out plan for raising us and they had the time to see it through.

Even though my parents pushed me hard, they gave me the freedom and support to make my own decisions. They provided me with options—and even at a very young age, they allowed me the opportunity to choose.

My parents held academics in high regard, and their policy was, as long as I had good grades, I could partake in music and sports, but only if I had good grades first. I got to attend the Escuela Libre de Música, a performing-arts high school in San Juan—Puerto Rico's version of *Fame*—where there ironically were no sports. But I learned a lot about music theory and am likely one of the few major league ballplayers who is familiar with twentieth-century composers like Hindemith and Stravinsky (but I confess I never played either in the clubhouse). It was there that I was introduced to jazz too. My brother and I both started composing there as well. I also listened to a lot of classic rock–and even though I played a traditional acoustic Spanish-style guitar, I can still hear and remember myself trying to play that classic rock song "More Than a Feeling." Ironically, it was by the band Boston.

My parents never saw me becoming either a professional athlete or a professional musician–they just wanted me to go to college and earn a degree. I suppose my mom envisioned me as a successful architect, engineer, doctor, or lawyer–but fate took a different path, as it just so happened that the New York Yankees organization came by and saw me play baseball when I was fifteen years old. The next year, I signed a contract with them–it was 1985 and I was but sixteen years old. I left home and brought my guitar with me. The beauty of it is that during the sixteen years I played with the Yankees, I never felt like I gave up music because I never envisioned making a living as a musician. But the first thing I did when I got into the major leagues was to head to a music store in Times Square and buy my very first electric guitar. It was a Fender Stratocaster.

The three of us–Bob, Dave, and I–share something else in common beyond music and baseball. The three of us are parents. We've talked about the experience of going to our children's recitals, competitions, and games (by the way, Dave's second passion is as a high-school-level umpire, and Bob's passed up some pretty heavy gigs to be sure he didn't miss any of his son Christopher's Little League games).

Early on, it's critical that parents provide a supportive environment for their children when they exhibit a natural disposition and interest in art or sport. There is nothing sadder than seeing parents lose proportion and sensibility when it comes to their child's Little League game or recital. The parent yelling at their child for forgetting to make the tag, or for not playing well at the recital or concert is indeed a sad sight.

Parents often start with good intentions–wanting the best for their children, but again: it's not the results they should be concerned with–it's instilling in their children the need for hard work and a positive attitude. When kids aren't having fun playing ball or music, something is clearly wrong.

Early on, it's important for parents to not focus on the mechanical and technical aspects of music or baseball–but it's very important that parents provide their children with a nurturing, supportive environment that cultivates a non-pressured, enthusiastic, respectful, and fun yet focused atmosphere. If you can give your children this–and let the results be what they may–you'll be giving them a gift of strength and courage throughout their lives.

Above all, inspire passion in your children through music, baseball, or wherever their interests lie. Ideally, a child should be attracted to an activity on their own–they shouldn't be told to practice. Ideally, it shouldn't even feel like it's practice in the mind of a child. Discovery is at the root of passion and lifelong learning.

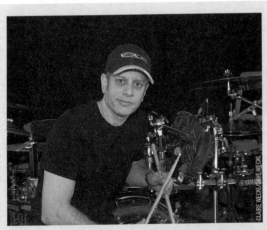

## RESPECT

by Dave Weckl, acclaimed jazz drummer who's performed with Bernie Williams, Paul Simon, Robert Plant, George Benson, the Brecker Brothers, and Chick Corea, among many others

Surprisingly, my dad probably pushed me more to be a baseball player than a musician! He was a baseball player himself and also a pianist, but he supported me in both. As a young ballplayer and musician, I grew up with admiration and respect for great ballplayers and musicians. There's this mutual admiration between professional ballplayers and musicians–each understands that it first takes a blessing of talent when you're very young. It also takes parents who can nurture and support that talent so that, when we're older, we can take advantage of it. While everyone grows up to be their own person, the fact is that we're all molded at an early age. The greatest gift parents can give young ballplayers and musicians is to encourage them to be mature and respectful at an early age. The more mature and respectful you are, the more you're going to learn. And by the same token, the more you practice and the harder you work, the better you will get!

# THE LOSS THAT WASN'T

by Bob Thompson, as published in *The New York Times*, June 13, 2010

A Sunday in May. I'm watching my son's Little League game at the ball field on the corner of 97th and Second. The third baseline is but a few feet away from the street.

It's the top of the fourth inning, and a kid hits a foul ball, but someone forgot to close the gate. The ball bounces onto the street just as a taxi driver, window rolled down, still driving, reaches out with his left hand and catches the ball on one hop.

Everyone breaks into applause and cheers for the driver. He smiles, one-arms the ball back onto the field and drives off.

Play resumes. My son's team loses, 10–6. Ten years from now he will have forgotten the loss, but he won't forget that taxi driver.

# Postscript
# The Sound Track
# of Summer

by Tim Wiles, baseball researcher and
author, Cooperstown, New York

In many modern ballparks, each time a hitter strolls to the plate or a pitcher warms up, he is accompanied by a personally selected theme song. While many fans have noticed this trend, few have thought of its deeper implications for popular culture. Nothing defines a culture at the popular level better than its music, something which almost everyone enjoys (try to find someone who doesn't like music on at least some level). Another great indicator of a society's cultural values and passions is its sports. So when Roger Clemens grooves to Elton John's "Rocket Man," or Al Leiter gets pumped while warming up to Springsteen's "Tenth Avenue Freeze Out," it is not just a fun moment in the ballpark; it also tells us something about these players, and more importantly, something about ourselves. This recent development is only the latest of dozens, if not hundreds, of connections between music and baseball.

Surveying the thick file of clippings labeled "music" at the Baseball Hall of Fame Library, we find many more. References to the giant Margaret and Franklin Steele sheet-music collection and to the now nine-disc strong *Diamond Cuts* baseball music compilations are side by side with other gems. There are so many connections between baseball and music, that it's safe to say there are two national pastimes!

The earliest two known baseball songs, "The Baseball Polka" and "Baseball Days," were written in 1858. The first ballpark organ was installed at Wrigley Field in 1941. Just five years later, the National League felt it necessary to ban the song "Three Blind Mice," after Ebbets Field organist Gladys Goodding made a habit of playing it after close calls that went against the Dodgers. The Brooklyn Sym-Phony was an inspired group of fans who serenaded the Ebbets Field crowd, without the benefit of formal musical training.

The Yankees have even inspired a Broadway musical, *Damn Yankees,* about the team that's so hard to beat, one's thoughts turn to desperate measures. There have been several teams with theme songs—the 1979 Pirates bonded over Sister Sledge's "We Are Family." The Yanks of 1940 liked "Roll Out the Barrel," and of course, the 2004 Red Sox breathed new life into "Tessie," the theme song of the old Royal Rooters as performed by the Dropkick Murphys.

The list of players with musical talent is quite long. Former Padre infielder Tim Flannery has released several country-folk CDs. Denny McLain played the organ, both in clubs and on his own records. Jack McDowell's second career is as a rock-and-roll guitarist with his band Stickfigure, and Tony Conigliaro released a few singles as a singer. Mudcat Grant has a band, and Bronson Arroyo released an album called *Covering the Bases.* And don't forget Deion Sanders's 1995 CD, *Prime Time.* And, of course, there's Bernie Williams.

In his wonderful 1989 book, *Everything Baseball,* James Mote  imagined an all-time all-star team of ballplayer/musicians: Maury Wills on the banjo, Carmen Fanzone on trumpet, Pepper Martin on guitar, Babe Ruth on the sax, Charlie Maxwell on drums, Bob Kennedy on xylophone, Joe Pepitone on harmonica, Frankie Pytlak on mandolin, and Denny McLain on organ.

"Take Me Out to the Ball Game" has been recorded by big league ballplayers twice (prior to Bernie Williams's recording of it), once by a quartet that featured Phil Rizzuto, Ralph Branca, Roy Campanella, and Tommy Henrich, in 1950. Braves pitcher Buzz Capra recorded a version in 1975. The song was also recorded by one umpire, Joe West (1984), and one owner, Bing Crosby, part owner of the Pirates, in 1960.

There are also many players who've been mentioned in popular songs, or who have had entire songs written about them, such as Bill Lee, immortalized in a song called "Bill

Lee" by the late Warren Zevon. Richie Allen got a poignant appreciation from folksinger Chuck Brodsky in his song "Letters in the Dirt." Vida Blue has a whole band named after him. Jimmy Buffett and Johnny Ramone are among the many musicians who've been great baseball fans. Emmylou Harris was recently quoted as saying: "Let's just say I'm a National League girl, because I don't believe in the designated hitter." Country legend Charley Pride played baseball in the Negro Leagues. Duke Ellington enjoyed the game as a young man. Carly Simon, who does a definitive version of "Take Me Out to the Ball Game" on the soundtrack to Ken Burns's baseball documentary, grew up in Stamford, Connecticut, where her parents were friends with Jackie and Rachel Robinson. Carly would often ride to Ebbets Field in Jackie's car, and would sit in the dugout before games.

The list of American musicians, songwriters, and composers who've written on the game is a Hall of Fame in itself: George M. Cohan, John Philip Sousa, Irving Berlin, Charles Ives, Frank Sinatra, Chuck Berry, Bob Dylan, John Fogerty, Jonathan Richman, Dave Frishberg, Paul Simon, Count Basie, Woody Guthrie, and Bruce Springsteen.

Writers have also gotten into the game, musically speaking. Ring Lardner wrote a bouncy little number called "Gee It's a Wonderful Game," in 1911. Peter Gammons is a well-known devotee of the independent music scene, as well as a songwriter and musician in his own right. Henry Chadwick, the father of baseball writing, also wrote and published approximately fifty instrumental compositions, according to new research by Cooperstown-based baseball historian Peter Nash, himself the former leader of a rap band called 3rd Bass, whose several baseball songs included one on Ted "Double Duty" Radcliffe, the recently deceased star of the Negro Leagues.

A surprising number of Hall of Famers have been deeply involved in music. According to former Hall of Fame historian Ken Smith, Frankie Frisch played the violin, Mickey Cochrane favored the saxophone, Waite Hoyt was a fine singer (and a painter too), and Bill Terry possessed a "clear-voiced baritone."

Terry Cashman's 1981 hit "Talkin' Baseball, Willie, Mickey, and the Duke," celebrated the golden era of both baseball in general, and center fielders in particular. At a time when fans were enduring the first major baseball strike, they enjoyed a bit of pure nostalgia for simpler times, thanks to Cashman's infectious melody and clear love for the game. Mays was mentioned in Bob Dylan's "I Shall Be Free," and also was the subject of the infectious "Say Hey (The Willie Mays Song)" by the Treniers. Mantle had his own musical tribute, Teresa Brewer's "I Love Mickey."

"Where have you gone, Joe DiMaggio?" asked Paul Simon poignantly in the song "Mrs. Robinson," and the great center fielder was also the subject of two songs: "Joltin' Joe DiMaggio" by Les Brown and his Band of Renown and "Joe DiMaggio Done It Again" by Woody Guthrie.

Irving Berlin's 1926 composition "Along Came Ruth" was one of a nearly dozen songs inspired by the Babe's home-run prowess. Ernie Harwell penned a 1974 tribute to Babe and his successor Hank Aaron, entitled "Move Over Babe, Here Comes Henry."

Like dozens of other ballplayers, including the Babe, Rube Marquard had a Vaudeville routine. He was also the subject of a popular song, "That Marquard Glide." Mike Schmidt, along with teammates Garry Maddox, Dave Cash, Larry Bowa, and Greg Luzinski, recorded "Phillies Fever" in 1976. Bob Dylan wrote an ode to Catfish Hunter in the 1970s, with the prophetic couplet, "Every season twenty wins/Gonna make the Hall of Fame."

There is an alternative rock band called Ty Cobb, whose sound has been described as "hard driven and purely American." Sounds like they picked a good name. Richie Ashburn's 1962 collision with Elia Chacon has resulted in another band name, the veteran New Jersey rockers known as Yo La Tengo, which is Spanish for "I got it," which Chacon yelled and Ashburn didn't understand, resulting in the collision. Songwriter Evan Johns has written "Bill Veeck the Baseball Man" about the great showman. And who can ever forget Stan Musial playing "Take Me Out to the Ball Game" on his harmonica, or Gary Carter singing "Oh Canada" at the induction ceremonies, let alone Johnny Bench's hilarious send-up of Harry Caray's singing? Hall of Famers have indeed made their marks in the world of music as well as in the game itself.

From 1858 to the present, there has been a strong relationship between our great game of baseball and the timeless world of music. For fans of both, there is far more than initially meets the eye, or, in this case, the ear.

*This essay originally appeared in* Baseball's Greatest Hit: The Story of Take Me Out to the Ballgame, *©2008 by Andy Strasberg, Bob Thompson, and Tim Wiles, reprinted by permission of Hal Leonard.*

## JEER HERE!

by Meagan Curtis

At the ballpark, the music of baseball is all around us, from the songs that energize the fans (and hopefully the team) to the taunts being spewed at the opposing team by the oaf a few rows away. Yes, you read that correctly: the loudmouth who is taunting the batter may be producing vocalizations that have strong links to music. From the time we are children, our taunts have a musical sing-song quality, and we actually use a vocal pitch pattern that is important in the musical communication of negative emotions. The childhood taunt, "Nyah-nyah," is generally said with the pitch pattern of a descending minor third. In Western music, the minor third is a defining feature of the minor mode, which is used to communicate negative emotions. What does this childhood taunt have to do with Yankees fans yelling, "Who's your daddy?" whenever Pedro Martinez takes the mound? The pitch pattern of this and other baseball taunts tends to be a minor third. To the chagrin of Red Sox fans, when Pedro had a rough start against the Yankees in 2004, he famously gave Yankees fans ammunition, saying, "What can I say? I tip my hat and call the Yankees my daddy." The next time Pedro took the mound against the Yankees, the New York fans greeted him by taunting, "Who's your daddy?" If you're from New York or Boston, you're probably familiar with this taunt and its pitch pattern. Minor thirds abound in baseball taunts, so much so that the fans don't need to say something incendiary to convey that they are taunting a player; the minor third carries the emotional message. For instance, Red Sox fans love to taunt Derek Jeter and Alex Rodriguez whenever they come up to bat. The next time you watch the Sox play the Yanks, listen carefully. You'll hear Sox fans yelling, "Jeee-ter" and "Aaaaa-Rod" in minor thirds. Will it sound like music to your ears? Only if you're a Red Sox fan.

## 5-0: OUR FIVE FAVORITE "BASEBALL" CONCERTS OF ALL TIME

by Bernie Williams, Dave Gluck, and Bob Thompson

I'd rather be a musician than a rock star.
–*George Harrison*

### The Beatles at Shea Stadium (August 15, 1965)

On that same evening, in another borough of New York City, the Yankees hosted the Kansas City Athletics in a doubleheader. The teams split the decision in front of a crowd of 21,441– less than half the audience who decided to see the Beatles perform at Shea Stadium.

### Jimi Hendrix at Woodstock (August 18, 1969)

On the day that Jimi Hendrix performed the "Star Spangled Banner" on an early Monday morning to a small, dwindling crowd at the end of the three-day Woodstock Festival, Hank Aaron appeared on the cover of *Sports Illustrated* with the headline "Henry Aaron whips Atlanta into its first pennant drive." William Leggett wrote in his magazine article, "For years Henry Aaron performed in comparative obscurity while compiling a record that makes him one of baseball's all-time hitters. Now, as Atlanta fights for a pennant, he finds he is famous at last."

### Simon and Garfunkel in Central Park (September 19, 1981)

Yankees fans in New York didn't need to choose between heading to the Bronx or to Central Park in Manhattan to see Simon and Garfunkel perform in this epic concert–the Yankees were on the road. That night, the Yanks played the

Red Sox at Fenway and lost, 8–5, in front of 32,620 fans. Simon and Garfunkel performed to a crowd that was slightly larger—over 500,000 people.

## Led Zeppelin's Three Nights at Madison Square Garden (July 27, 28, and 29, 1973)

On July 27, 1973, the Yanks outlasted Jim Colborn and the Milwaukee Brewers in twelve innings, 1–0, as the game was won on a Thurman Munson single. It was in that same year that the old Yankee Stadium on the south side of 161st Street was closed and renovated.

## Pink Floyd's *The Wall* at Earls Court Arena (June 17, 1981)

The last live performance of this unprecedented, infamous tour was on June 17, 1981, at London's Earls Court Arena. Unlike the choice Yankees fans had to make on August 15, 1965, between a Beatles concert at Shea or a ball game at Yankee Stadium, the last *The Wall* concert didn't present Yankees fans with a tough decision-making dilemma—not only was Pink Floyd performing in London on this night, but Major League Baseball was in the midst of a mid-season strike that began five days earlier, on June 12.

# Acknowledgments

BERNIE: I'd like to thank my family, especially my wife, Waleska, and my children, Bernie Jr., Beatriz, and Bianca, my brother, Hiram, and of course my parents. I'd also like to thank all those coaches and music teachers in my life who have supported and inspired me—especially my first Little League coach, Jorge Lopez; Roberto Rivera, the Yankees scout who signed me; and finally, Eduardo Flores, my first guitar teacher.

DAVE: I would like to give heartfelt thanks to my loving and supportive wife, Nicole, and my three wonderful sons, Julian, Noah, and Jasper.

BOB: I'd like to thank my family—my sister, Linda, my brother, Mitchell, my dear aunt, Barbara, and finally my two wonderful children—Christopher and Emily, who have brought more joy to my life than the worlds of music and baseball combined.

The three of us would like to collectively acknowledge:

Paul Simon, to whom we owe a special debt of gratitude. In the midst of a new album and a tour, Paul graciously took time out to write the foreword to our book. It's impossible to conceive of a book about music and baseball without Paul Simon in it—thank you, Paul.

Steve Fortunato, our dear friend and colleague. This book would not have been possible without Steve's unwavering support, time, and effort. Thank you, Fortch!

The many people who gave graciously of their time and talents:

Marty Appel, Kenny Aronoff, Bonnie Bernstein, Yogi Berra,

Ken Burns, Richie Cannata, John Cerullo, Chris Clark, Todd Coolman, Bob Costas, Meagan Curtis, Juanita DeSilva, Jon Faddis, Mike Francesa, Tim Gallwey, Barry Green, Don Greene, Randy Grossman, Fred Hand, Loren Harriet, Ariele Goldman Hecht, Jeff Idelson, Timothy Johnson, Michael Kay, Marybeth Keating, Steven Lubin, Pete Malinverni, Keith Mardak, Bill Menzel, Richie Morales, Sweeny Murti, Alan Nathan, Tim Parsaca, Nalina Riggio, Cal Ripken, Jr., Heather Saunders, Marie Sciangula, Wes Seeley, Weston Sprott, John Sterling, Andy Strasberg, Fred Sturm, Joe Torre, Debbie Tymon, Suzyn Waldman, Dave Weckl, Tim Wiles, Dave Winfield, and Kristi Zimmerman.

# Bibliography

"100 Most Memorable Moments: Jeter's backhand flip rescues Yankees." *ESPN.* http://sports.espn.go.com.

"50 Great Moments in Jazz: Keith Jarrett's *The Köln Concert,*" January 31, 2011. http://www.guardian.co.uk.

"Aguinaldo." *Wikipedia.* http://en.wikipedia.org.

Alda, Alan. "The creative is the place where no one else has ever been . . ." http://www.famous-quotes.com.

Andersen, Mark. *Doing Sport Psychology.* 1st ed. Human Kinetics, 2000.

Angell, Roger. *The Summer Game.* New York: Viking Press, 1972.

Anshel, Mark H. *Sport Psychology: From Theory to Practice.* 4th ed. Benjamin Cummings, 2002.

Appel, Marty. *Munson: The Life and Death of a Yankee Captain.* New York: Doubleday, 2009.

———. *Now Pitching for the Yankees: Spinning the News for Mickey, Billy, and George.* Kingston, NY: Total/Sports Illustrated, 2001.

———. *Slide, Kelly, Slide: The Wild Life and Times of Mike King Kelly.* 1st ed. New York: The Scarecrow Press, 1999.

Aronoff, Kenny. Interview with the authors, October 2010.

Barnes, Craig. "Loretta Adjusting to Boston." *Sun Sentinel,* March 16, 2003. http://articles.sun-sentinel.com.

Barrell, James J., and David Ryback. *Psychology of Champions: How to Win at Sports and Life with the Focus Edge of Super-Athletes.* Praeger, 2008.

*Baseball.* PBS, 1994.

"The Baseball Music Project." http://www.baseballmusicproject.com.

"Baseball's Sad Lexicon." *Wikipedia.* http://en.wikipedia.org.

Basinski, Eddie. *Baseball Digest.* Lakeside Publishing Co., 1949.

Bassham, Lanny R. *With Winning in Mind: The Mental Management System.* New edition. Book-partners, 1996.

"Battle Rap." *Wikipedia.* http://en.wikipedia.org.

Baum, Kenneth. *The Mental Edge.* 1st ed. Perigee Trade, 1999.

Becker, Boris. "I love the winning, I can take the losing, but most of all I love to play." http://www.dictionary-quotes.com.

"Bernie Williams." *Wikipedia.* http://en.wikipedia.org.

"Bernie Williams Statistics and History." *Baseball-Reference.com.* http://www.baseball-reference.com.

Berra, Yogi. "Little League baseball is a very good thing because it keeps the parents off the streets." http://www.dictionary-quotes.com.

Bishop, Daniel T. "A Grounded Theory of Young Tennis Players' Use of Music to Manipulate Emotional State." *Journal of Sport & Exercise Psychology* 29, no. 5 (October 2007): 584–607. http://journals.humankinetics.com.

Bishop, Daniel T., and Costas I Karageorghis. "Effects of Musically-Induced Emotions on Choice Reaction Time Performance." *The Sport Psychologist* 23, no. 1 (March 2009): 59–76. http://journals.humankinetics.com.

Blatt, Howard. *This Championship Season: The Incredible Story of the 1998 New York Yankees' Record-Breaking 125 Win Year.* New York: Pocket Books, 1998.

Bondy, Flip. "Pedro Martinez's Six Innings Deliver Big Hope for October." *New York Daily News.* September 16, 2007. http://www.nydailynews.com.

Boutcher, Stephen H., and Michele Trenske. "The Effects of Sensory Deprivation and Music on Perceived Exertion and Affect During Exercise." *Journal of Sport & Exercise Psychology* 12,

# BIBLIOGRAPHY

no. 2 (June 1990): 167–178. http://journals.humankinetics.com.

Boyd, Jenny. *Musicians in Tune: 75 Contemporary Musicians Discuss the Creative Process*. Fireside, 1992.

Brooks, Garth. "As a kid, before I could play music, I remember baseball being the one thing that could always make me happy." http://www.brainyquote.com.

Burns, Ken. *Baseball (10th Inning)*. PBS, 2010.

–––. *Baseball (Innings 1–9)*. PBS, 2004.

Burton, Damon, and Thomas Raedeke. *Sport Psychology for Coaches*. 1st ed. Human Kinetics, 2008.

Butler, Richard J. *Sports Psychology in Performance*. 1st ed. A Hodder Arnold Publication, 1997.

Canfield, Jack, Mark Victor Hansen, Chrissy Donnelly, and Mark Donnelly. *Chicken Soup for the Baseball Fan's Soul: Inspirational Stories of Baseball, Big-League Dreams and the Game of Life*. HCI, 2001.

Cannata, Richie. Interview with the authors, October 2010.

Carranco, Lynwood. "Joe Oeschger Remembers." *SABR Baseball Research Journal Archives* (1980). http://research.sabr.org.

Carse, James P. *Finite and Infinite Games: A Vision of Life as Play and Possibility*. Ballantine Books, 1987.

Caruso, Andrew. *Sports Psychology Basics*. Reedswain, 2004.

Clark, Chris. Interview with the authors, October 2010.

"The Concert in Central Park." *Wikipedia*. http://en.wikipedia.org.

Cox, Richard. *Sport Psychology: Concepts and Applications*. 6th ed. McGraw-Hill Humanities/Social Sciences/Languages, 2006.

Coyle, Daniel. *The Talent Code: Greatness Isn't Born. It's Grown. Here's How*. 1st ed. Bantam, 2009.

Craig, Gary. *EFT for Sports Performance*. Energy Psychology Press, 2010.

Deutsch, Diana. The Psychology of Music. 2nd ed. Academic Press, 1998.

Donnelly, Chris. *Baseball's Greatest Series: Yankees, Mariners, and the 1995 Matchup That Changed History*. New Brunswick, NJ: Rivergate Books/Rutgers University Press, 2010.

Dorfman, H. A. *Coaching the Mental Game: Leadership Philosophies and Strategies for Peak Performance in Sports and Everyday Life*. Taylor Trade Publishing, 2005.

–––. *The Mental Game of Baseball: A Guide to Peak Performance*. 3rd ed. Diamond Communications, 2002.

Dosil, Joaquin. *The Sport Psychologist's Handbook: A Guide for Sport-Specific Performance Enhancement*. 1st ed. Wiley, 2005.

Dubow, Josh. "Yanks Return Home; Lose Game, but Win Division." The Associated Press, September 26, 2001. http://nl.newsbank.com.

Early, Gerald. "Burns Strikes a Jazz Chord." *CBS Sunday Morning–CBS News*. http://www.cbsnews.com.

Edison, Thomas. "Nearly every man who develops an idea . . ." http://thinkexist.com.

Emerson, Ralph Waldo. "People succeed when they realize that their failures are the preparation for their victories." http://www.wow4u.com.

Ericsson, Anders K., Neil Charness, Paul J. Feltovich, and Robert R. Hoffman. *The Cambridge Handbook of Expertise and Expert Performance*. 1st ed. Cambridge University Press, 2006.

Ericsson, Anders K., Michael J. Prietula, and Edward T. Cokely. "The Making of an Expert." *Harvard Business Review*, July–August 2007. http://hbr.org.

Etnier, Jennifer L. *Bring Your "A" Game: A Young Athlete's Guide to Mental Toughness*. The University of North Carolina Press, 2009.

Faddis, Jon. Interview with the authors, December 2010.

Fellowship of Christian Athletes. *Teamwork: The Heart and Soul in Sports*. Regal, 2009.

Fenger, Hans. "The Langley Schools Music Project: Innocence and Despair." http://www.keyofz.com.

Fish, Joel. *101 Ways to Be a Terrific Sports Parent : Making Athletics a Positive Experience for Your Child*. Original. Fireside, 2003.

# BIBLIOGRAPHY

Fonseca-Wollheim, Corinna. "A Jazz Night to Remember." wsj.com, October 11, 2008, sec. Masterpiece. http://online.wsj.com.

"Frank Zappa: Irregular Rhythmic Groupings." http://www.zappa-analysis.com.

Frith, Fred. "Improvised music involves a lot of intuition and I like developing intuition." http://www.brainyquote.com.

Galenson, David. "The Greatest Artists of the Twentieth Century." National Bureau of Economic Research Working Paper Series, No. 11899 (December 2005). http://www.nber.org.

Gallucci, Nicholas T. *Sport Psychology: Performance Enhancement, Performance Inhibition, Individuals, and Teams*. 1st ed. Psychology Press, 2008.

Gallwey, W. Timothy. *The Inner Game of Tennis*. 1st ed. New York: Random House, 1974.

Gardner, Frank, and Zella E. Moore. *Clinical Sport Psychology*. 1st ed. Human Kinetics, 2005.

———. *The Psychology of Enhancing Human Performance: The Mindfulness-Acceptance-Commitment Approach*. 1st ed. Springer Publishing Company, 2007.

Gawain, Shakti. *Creative Visualization*. 1st ed. Berkeley, CA: Whatever Pub, 1978.

Giamatti, A. Bartlett. *A Great and Glorious Game: Baseball Writings of A. Bartlett Giamatti*. 1st ed. Chapel Hill, NC: Algonquin Books, 1998.

Gill, Diane L., and Lavon Williams. *Psychological Dynamics of Sport and Exercise*. 3rd ed. Human Kinetics, 2008.

Gladwell, Malcolm. *Outliers: The Story of Success*. 1st ed. Little, Brown and Company, 2008.

Glanz, James. "The Crack of the Bat: Acoustics Takes on the Sound of Baseball." *The New York Times*, June 26, 2001, sec. Science. http://www.nytimes.com.

Goode, Michael I. *Stage Fright in Music Performance and Its Relationship to the Unconscious*. 2nd ed. Trumpetworks Press, 2003.

Gordon, Stewart. *Mastering the Art of Performance: A Primer for Musicians*. Oxford University Press, 2010.

Green, Barry. *The Inner Game of Music*. Garden City, NY: Anchor Press/Doubleday, 1986.

———. *The Mastery of Music: Ten Pathways to True Artistry*. 1st ed. New York: Broadway Books, 2003.

Greene, Don. *Audition Success: An Olympic Sports Psychologist Teaches Performing Artists How to Win*. New York: Routledge, 2001.

———. *Fight Your Fear and Win: Seven Skills for Performing Your Best Under Pressure: At Work, in Sports, on Stage*. New York: Broadway Books, 2001.

———. *Focused Performances: A Journey of Understanding*. San Diego, CA: ProMind Music, 2011.

———. *Performance Success: Performing Your Best Under Pressure*. New York: Routledge, 2001.

Grimes, Andrea. "Blow Average: You Could Be a Star . . . but Please Don't Try." *Dallas Observer*, April 26, 2007. http://www.dallasobserver.com.

Hackfort, Dieter, and Charles D. Spielberger. *Anxiety in Sports: An International Perspective*. New edition. Taylor & Francis, 1990.

Haime, John. *You Are a Contender!: Build Emotional Muscle to Perform Better and Achieve More in Business, Sports and Life*. Morgan James Publishing, 2009.

Hall, Donald. "There's a lot of wonderful stillness in baseball that I love." https://journals.ku.edu.

Hallam, Susan, Ian Cross, and Michael Thaut. *Oxford Handbook of Music Psychology*. Oxford University Press, 2009.

Hand, Fred. Interview with the authors, October 2010.

Hardy, Lew, Graham Jones, and Daniel Gould. *Understanding Psychological Preparation for Sport: Theory and Practice of Elite Performers*. Wiley, 1996.

Harré, Rom, Siu-Lan Tan, and Peter Pfordresher. *Psychology of Music: From Sound to Significance*. 1st ed. Psych Press US, 2010.

Harrison, George. "I'd rather be a musician than a rock star." http://www.imdb.com.

Hays, Kate F. *Performance Psychology in Action: A Casebook for Working with Athletes, Performing Artists, Business Leaders, and Professionals in High-Risk Occupations*. 1st ed. American Psychological Association (APA), 2009.

Hemmings, Brian, and Tim Holder. *Applied Sport Psychology: A Case-Based Approach*. 1st ed.

# BIBLIOGRAPHY

Wiley, 2009.

Heuschkel, David. "1999: A Look Back." *Hartford Courant*, March 29, 2000. http://articles.courant.com.

Hill, Karen Lee. *Frameworks for Sport Psychologists: Enhancing Sport Performance*. 1st ed. Human Kinetics, 2000.

Hodges, Donald A. *Handbook of Music Psychology*. 2nd ed. MMB Music, 1996.

Hodges, Donald, and David Conrad Sebald. *Music in the Human Experience: An Introduction to Music Psychology*. Routledge, 2010.

Humphries, Rolfe. "Polo Grounds." *In Collected Poems of Rolfe Humphries*. Indiana University Press, 1966.

Huron, David. *Sweet Anticipation: Music and the Psychology of Expectation*. The MIT Press, 2008.

Jackson, Susan, and Mihaly Csikszentmihalyi. *Flow in Sports: The Keys to Optimal Experiences and Performances*. 1st ed. Human Kinetics, 1999.

Jagger, Mick. "You can play music forever. It's not like playing baseball." http://www.quotesdaddy.com.

Johnson, Magic. "Even as a fierce competitor I try to smile." http://www.thefamousquotations.com.

Johnson, Timothy A. *Baseball and the Music of Charles Ives: A Proving Ground*. Lanham, MD: Scarecrow Press, 2004.

Jowett, Sophia, and David Lavallee. *Social Psychology in Sport*. 1st ed. Human Kinetics, 2006.

"Jumpin Jack Flash." ABKCO Music Inc., 1968. http://repertoire.bmi.com.

Karageorghis, Costas I, and Denis A. Mouzourides. "Psychophysical and Ergogenic Effects of Synchronous Music During Treadmill Walking." *Journal of Sport & Exercise Psychology* 31, no. 1 (February 2009): 18–36. http://journals.humankinetics.com.

Karageorghis, Costas, and David-Lee Priest. "Music in Sport and Exercise: An Update on Research and Application." *The Sport Journal* 11, no. 3 (Summer 2008). http://www.thesportjournal.org.

Karageorghis, Costas, and Peter Terry. *Inside Sport Psychology*. 1st ed. Human Kinetics, 2010.

Kernan, Kevin. *Bernie Williams: Quiet Superstar*. Baseball Superstars Series 5. Champaign, IL: Sports Pub, 1999.

Keyes, Ralph. *The Quote Verifier: Who Said What, Where, and When*. Macmillan, 2006. http://books.google.com.

Kinsella, W. P. *Shoeless Joe*. 1st ed. Mariner Books, 1999.

Klickstein, Gerald. *The Musician's Way: A Guide to Practice, Performance, and Wellness*. Oxford University Press, 2009.

Kohut, Daniel L. *Musical Performance: Learning Theory and Pedagogy*. Stipes Publishing, LLC, 1992.

Kornspan, Alan. *Fundamentals of Sport and Exercise Psychology*. Human Kinetics, 2009.

Lambert, Charles. *Your Inner Edge!* Trafford Publishing, 2006.

Langley Schools Music Project. *Innocence & Despair*. Bar/None Records, 2001.

Lardon, Michael. *Finding Your Zone: Ten Core Lessons for Achieving Peak Performance in Sports and Life*. 1st ed. Perigee Trade, 2008.

Lasser, Fred Borden, Jeri Edwards, Dr. Eric S. *Sport Psychology Library: Bowling*. Fitness Information Technology, 2006.

Leavy, Jane, and OverDrive, Inc. *The Last Boy: Mickey Mantle and the End of America's Childhood*. New York: Harper, 2010.

Lehmann, Andreas C., John A. Sloboda, and Robert H. Woody. *Psychology for Musicians: Understanding and Acquiring the Skills*. 1st ed. Oxford University Press, 2007.

Lennon, John, and Paul McCartney. "Yesterday." Northern Songs, Ltd., 1965.

LeShan, Lawrence. *How to Meditate: A Guide to Self-Discovery*. 1st ed. Little, Brown and Company, 1999.

LeUnes, Arnold. *Sport Psychology*. 4th ed. Psychology Press, 2008.

Levitin, Daniel J. *This Is Your Brain on Music: The Science of a Human Obsession*. Plume, 2006.

# BIBLIOGRAPHY

Loehr, James E. *The New Toughness Training for Sports: Mental, Emotional, and Physical Conditioning from One of the World's Premier Sports Psychologists*. Plume, 1995.

"Los Panchos." *Wikipedia*. http://en.wikipedia.org.

Mack, Gary, and David Casstevens. *Mind Gym: An Athlete's Guide to Inner Excellence*. 1st ed. McGraw-Hill, 2002.

Madden, Bill, and OverDrive, Inc. *Steinbrenner: The Last Lion of Baseball*. 1st ed. New York: Harper, 2010.

Maiman, Bruce. "The Conversation: Music and Its Transformative Power." *Sacramento Bee*. Sacramento, CA., February 13, 2011, sec. Opinion. http://www.sacbee.com.

Maltz, Maxwell. *Psycho-Cybernetics, A New Way to Get More Living Out of Life*. 7th ed. Pocket, 1989.

Meyer, Leonard B. *Emotion and Meaning in Music*. University of Chicago Press, 1961.

Meyer, Urban. "I have yet to be in a game where luck was involved . . ." http://www.gatortailgating.com.

Mills, Cliff. *Bernie Williams*. New York: Chelsea House, 2007.

Morales, Richie. Interview with the authors, October 2010.

Moran, Aidan P., and Aidan Moran. *The Psychology of Concentration in Sport Performers: A Cognitive Analysis*. 1st ed. Psychology Press, 1999.

Murphy, Shane. *The Sport Psych Handbook*. 1st ed. Human Kinetics, 2004.

Murray, Jim. Lou Gehrig: The Official Web Site. http://www.lougehrig.com.

Muskat, Carrie. *Bernie Williams*. Latinos in Baseball Series. Childs, MD: Mitchell Lane, 2000.

Nachmanovitch, Stephen. *Free Play: Improvisation in Life and Art*. Tarcher, 1991.

Nideffer, Robert M. A.C.T., *Attention Control Training: How to Get Control of Your Mind Through Total Concentration*. Wideview Books, 1979.

———. *An Athlete's Guide to Mental Training*. Human Kinetics Publishers, 1985.

———. *How to Put Anxiety Behind You*. Stein & Day Pub, 1978.

———. *The Inner Athlete*. Thomas Y. Crowell, 1986.

———. *Psyched to Win*. Human Kinetics Publishers, 1992.

"Ode to the Hot Dog." MLB.com. http://www.mlb.com.

Orlick, Terry. *In Pursuit of Excellence*. 4th ed. Human Kinetics, 2007.

Ortiz, John M. *The Tao of Music: Sound Psychology*. Weiser Books, 1997.

Panchos, Trio Los. *Trio Los Panchos*. Hal Leonard Corporation, 1999.

Paper, Lewis J. *Perfect: Don Larsen's Miraculous World Series Game and the Men Who Made It Happen*. New York: New American Library, 2009.

Pargman, David. *Managing Performance Stress: Models and Methods*. 1st ed. Routledge, 2006.

Parncutt, Richard, and Gary McPherson. *The Science and Psychology of Music Performance: Creative Strategies for Teaching and Learning*. Oxford University Press, 2002.

Patel, Aniruddh D. *Music, Language, and the Brain*. 1st ed. Oxford University Press, 2010.

Perlis, Alan J. "Perlisisms–Epigrams in Programming." http://www.cs.yale.edu.

Philadelphia Orchestra. *Romance*. Quartz Music Ltd, 2007.

Plato. *The Republic*. Translated by Benjamin Jowett. New York: The Modern Library, 1941.

Porter, Kay. *The Mental Athlete*. 1st ed. Human Kinetics, 2003.

Powell, John. *How Music Works: The Science and Psychology of Beautiful Sounds, from Beethoven to the Beatles and Beyond*. Little, Brown and Company, 2010.

Raalte, Judy L. Van, and Britton W. Brewer. *Exploring Sport and Exercise Psychology*. 2nd ed. American Psychological Association (APA), 2002.

Rendl, Maria, and Attila Szabo. "Performance Enhancement with Music in Rowing Sprint." *The Sport Psychologist* 22, no. 2 (June 2008): 175–182. http://journals.humankinetics.com.

Revesz, Geza. *Introduction to the Psychology of Music*. Dover Publications, 2001.

Robinson, Jackie. "A life is not important except in the impact it has on other lives." http://www.baseball-almanac.com.

Robinson, Phil Alden. *Field of Dreams*. Universal Studios, 2006.

Robson, Kenneth S., and David Halberstam. *In A Great and Glorious Game: Baseball Writings of A. Bartlett Giamatti*. 1st ed. Algonquin Books, 1998.

# BIBLIOGRAPHY

Rockne, Knute. "The secret is to work less as individuals and more as a team." http://www. great-motivational-quotes.com.

Sacks, Oliver. *Musicophilia: Tales of Music and the Brain.* Revised and expanded edition. Vintage, 2008.

Selk, Jason. *10-Minute Toughness: The Mental Training Program for Winning Before the Game Begins.* 1st ed. McGraw-Hill, 2008.

Shakespeare, William. "The circumstances of the world are so variable . . ." http://www.quotesdaddy.com.

Simon, Carly. *Anticipation.* C'est Music, 1971.

Simon, Paul. "I always get very calm with baseball." http://www.brainyquote.com.

Singletary, Michael. "Do you know what my favorite part of the game is? The opportunity to play." http://www.goodquotes.com.

Smith, Daniel, and Michael Bar-Eli. *Essential Readings in Sport and Exercise Psychology.* 1st ed. Human Kinetics, 2007.

Smith, Leif H., and Todd M. Kays. *Sports Psychology for Dummies.* 1st ed. For Dummies, 2010.

Snyder, Eldon E. "Responses to Musical Selections and Sport: An Auditory Elicitation Approach." *Sociology of Sport Journal* 10, no. 2 (June 1993): 168–182. http://journals.humankinetics.com.

Stewart, Mark. *Bernie Williams: Quiet Leader.* New York: Children's Press, 1998.

Storr, Anthony. *Music and the Mind.* Ballantine Books, 1993.

Strasberg, Andy, Bob Thompson, and Tim Wiles. *Baseball's Greatest Hit: The Story of "Take Me Out to the Ball Game."* New York: Hal Leonard Corporation, 2008.

Summers, Adam. "Battered Expectations: Do Baseballs Obey the Conventional Laws of Physics?." *Natural History Magazine,* July–August (2008). http://www.naturalhistorymag. com.

"Tampa Bay Devil Rays vs. New York Yankees." *ESPN,* September 25, 2001. http://scores.espn. go.com.

Tan, Siu-Lan, Peter Pfordresher, and Rom Harré. *Psychology of Music: From Sound to Significance.* 1st ed. Psychology Press, 2010.

Taylor, Jim, and Gregory Wilson. *Applying Sport Psychology: Four Perspectives.* 1st ed. Human Kinetics, 2005.

Temperley, David. *Music and Probability.* The MIT Press, 2010.

Templin , David P., and Ralph A. Vernacchia. "The Effect of Highlight Music Videotapes Upon the Game Performance of Intercollegiate Basketball Players." *The Sport Psychologist* 9, no. 1 (March 1995): 41–50. http://journals.humankinetics.com.

Tenenbaum, Gershon. *The Practice of Sport Psychology.* Fitness Information Technology, 2001.

Thompson, William Forde. *Music, Thought, and Feeling: Understanding the Psychology of Music.* 1st ed. Oxford University Press, 2008.

Torre, Joe. *The Yankee Years.* 1st ed. New York: Anchor Books, 2010.

Townshend, Peter. "Won't Get Fooled Again." ABKCO Music Inc., 1971.

Truman, Harry S. "It is amazing what can be accomplished when it doesn't matter who gets the credit." http://www.quotesdaddy.com.

Tsvetaeva, Marina. "A deception that elevates us is dearer than a host of low truths." http:// www.finestquotes.com.

Uecker, Bob. "I knew when my career was over. In 1965 my baseball card came out with no picture." http://www.brainyquote.com.

Various Artists. *Baseball's Greatest Hits.* Rhino/Wea, 1992.

– – –. *Baseball's Greatest Hits II: Let's Play.* Rhino/Wea, 1992.

Vaughn, Stephen L. *Encyclopedia of American Journalism.* CRC Press, 2008.

Waldman, Scott. "Billie Holiday and Lester Young: A Musical Romance." PopMatters. http:// www.popmatters.com.

Waldman, Suzyn. Interview with the authors, January 2011.

Wann, Daniel L. *Sport Psychology.* Prentice Hall, 1996.

Ward, Geoffrey C. *Baseball: An Illustrated History.* Updated ed. New York: Alfred A. Knopf, 2010.

# BIBLIOGRAPHY

Ward, Geoffrey C., and Ken Burns. *Jazz: A History of America's Music.* 1st ed. Knopf, 2000.

Weinberg, Robert, and Daniel Gould. *Foundations of Sport and Exercise Psychology.* 4th ed. Human Kinetics, 2006.

Werner, Kenny. *Effortless Mastery: Liberating the Master Musician Within.* Jamey Aebersold, 1996.

Whiting, Robert. "Contract Loophole Opened Door for Nomo's Jump." *The Japan Times Online,* October 10, 2010. http://search.japantimes.co.jp.

Wickens, Christopher D., and Justin G. Hollands. *Engineering Psychology and Human Performance.* 3rd ed. Prentice Hall, 1999.

Wiles, Andy, Bob Thompson, and Andy Strasberg. "The Soundtrack of Summer." In *Baseball's Greatest Hit: The Story of "Take Me Out to the Ball Game,"* 101–105. New York: Hal Leonard Corporation, 2008.

Williamon, Aaron. *Musical Excellence: Strategies and Techniques to Enhance Performance.* 1st ed. Oxford University Press, 2004.

Williams, Bernie. *Moving Forward.* Compact Disc. Reform Records/Rock Ridge Music, 2009.

–––. *The Journey Within.* Compact Disc. New York: GRP Records, 2003.

Williams, Don, Jr. "Despair is most often the offspring of ill-preparedness." http://www.examiner.com.

Williams, Jean. *Applied Sport Psychology: Personal Growth to Peak Performance.* 2nd ed. Saunders College Publishing/Harcourt Brace, 1986.

–––. *Applied Sport Psychology: Personal Growth to Peak Performance.* 6th ed. McGraw-Hill Humanities/Social Sciences/Languages, 2009.

Wilson, Earl. "For the parents of a Little Leaguer, a baseball game is simply a nervous breakdown divided into innings." http://espn.go.com.

Winfield, Dave. "My fondest memories of the game are as a kid playing catch with my brother . . ." Presented at The Baseball Music Project.

Witnauer, William D., Richard G. Rogers, and Jarron M. Saint Onge. "Major League Career Length in the 20th Century." *Popular Research and Policy Review* 26, no. 4 (2007): 371–386.

*Yankeeography.* Distributed by Hart Sharp Video, 2004.

Young, Geoff. "Epic Pitchers' Duels." http://www.hardballtimes.com.

Zappa, Frank. "Some people crave baseball–I find this unfathomable." *Wikipedia.* http://en.wikiquote.org.

Zimmerman, Barry J., and Dale H. Schunk. *Handbook of Self-Regulation of Learning and Performance.* Routledge, 2011.

# About the Authors

Originally from Utica, New York, **Dave Gluck** is a professor of studio composition at Purchase College, State University of New York. As a founding member of Rhythm & Brass, he has toured the globe as a percussionist, and has also appeared with numerous orchestras, including Phoenix, Colorado Springs, Oregon, Tucson, the Boston Pops Esplanade touring ensemble, and the United States Air Force Orchestra in Washington, D.C., to name but just a few. An acclaimed composer and arranger, his music has been featured in *Jazz Player Magazine* and on BET Network and NPR's *Fresh Air*, among others. Rhythm & Brass, acclaimed by *Entertainment Weekly* and the *American Record Guide*, has produced six recordings. *More Money Jungle . . . Ellington Explorations* (Koch Jazz) was named by *The New York Times* as "Album of the Week" in May 1999. A former member of Dallas Brass and a founder of Madera Vox, David is a Yamaha, Zildjian, and Innovative performing artist. Most recently, as a featured percussionist, David recorded with Bernie Williams on *Moving Forward*, for which the live performance was broadcast on the YES Network. He received his bachelor's degree in music from Ithaca College, was a teaching assistant at the University of North Texas, and earned his MM in studio composition from Purchase College.

Two-time Grammy-nominated producer and musician, **Bob Thompson** has toured and performed with such artists as the Moody Blues, Yes, Chuck Mangione, the Temptations, the Four Tops, Tony Bennett, Frank Sinatra, and Cab Calloway, as well as conducting the Chicago, Seattle, Detroit, San Diego, Houston, and Phoenix Symphonies, among others. Together with Hall of Famer Dave Winfield, Bob is the founder and creator of The Baseball Music Project, a multimedia series of concerts that celebrate the history of baseball through music and imagery. He's appeared on CBS's *Sun-

*day Morning* with Charles Osgood, where he talked about the project and his book, *Baseball's Greatest Hit: The Story of "Take Me Out to the Ball Game,"* for which Carly Simon wrote the foreword and Commissioner of Baseball Bud Selig wrote the introduction. Bob has served as dean of music at Purchase College, received the University of South Florida's Distinguished Alumni Award in 2005, and holds a doctorate in music from the Eastman School of Music, University of Rochester. He is originally from Hawthorne, New York, the final resting place of Babe Ruth.

Originally from Puerto Rico, **Bernie Williams** attended the Escuela Libre de Música, a performing-arts high school in San Juan, where he studied guitar, composition, and music theory while also showing prowess on the field as a baseball player. On his seventeenth birthday, he signed with the New York Yankees, where he played for sixteen years. During that time, he garnered four World Series rings, a Gold Glove, a batting title, and was a five-time All-Star player. His guitar always with him. Bernie continued to hone his musical skills during his baseball career, going on to record his first album, *The Journey Within*, in 2003, featuring such musicians as David Benoit, Ruben Blades and Béla Fleck. His second album, *Moving Forward*, released in 2009, garnered a Latin Grammy nomination and featured collaborative tracks with Bruce Springsteen, Patti Scialfa, Jon Secada, and Dave Koz. Bernie continues to tour and perform with his band and has appeared with musicians such as Paul Simon, Bruce Springsteen, Garth Brooks, Basia, and others. He is actively involved with numerous charitable organizations, including Hillside Food Outreach.

We've prepared a live program in which the three of us give a presentation, talk, and demonstration, followed by an audience discussion about *Rhythms of the Game* and the parallels between music and baseball. If you're interested in having us present this program at your school, organization, or event, please contact us at rhythmsofthegame@gmail.com or visit us on Facebook at www.facebook.com/rhythmsofthegame.